To Linda —

for the future!

J.

3/61/00

D1013809

VINTAGE PEOPLE

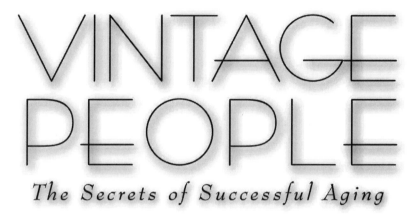

VINTAGE PEOPLE

The Secrets of Successful Aging

JERRY L. OLD, M.D.

PATHWAY PUBLISHING
Arkansas City, Kansas

Copyright © 2000 by Jerry L. Old, M.D.
All rights reserved.

ISBN 0-9677709-0-4

Printed in the United States of America
Published by Pathway Publishing
Route #2 Box 277 Arkansas City, Kansas 67005

Editing and page design by Griffith Publishing
Cover design by Griffith Anderson Design

DEDICATION

To all my patients, teachers, and friends
who have taught me about medicine and
about life.

TABLE OF CONTENTS

ACKNOWLEDGMENTS

I am greatly indebted to my secretary, my research assistant, my office manager, my consultant, my counselor, my psychiatrist, my nurse, my cook, my cheerleader, my best friend, my lover, and the most positive person I have ever known—they are all the same person—my wife Kristi. Without her I would never have even started on such a huge project.

Also, I want to thank my partners for taking up the slack while I was involved in researching and writing this book. During my preoccupation with writing, my children—Brandon (who now enjoys greater life with our Lord), Aaron, Allison, and Susan—saw less of me. A special thanks to those others who have encouraged me including my good friend Bill Bowles, whom I would like to emulate; Dottie Walters, the grand lady of public speaking; my coach Sandi Bigelow; Peter Lowe, the greatest encourager in the world; Senator Bob Dole, a remarkable "Vintage Person;" Joyce Griffith, for her astute editing skills; and all those I have met through their contributions to geriatric medicine.

Of course, tremendous thanks must go to the thousands of patients who have allowed me into their lives and have taught me the "art" of medicine over the years. However, the real stars of this book are the "Vintage People" who shared their ideas and secrets about what they are doing right in their lives that has allowed them to lead a long and successful existence. I stand in awe of their wisdom!

INTRODUCTION

I am a Board Certified Family Physician who has been in practice in a rural area of Kansas for twenty years. I am not an academician. I am a real-life, in-the-trenches rural doctor who still makes house calls, gets a lot of night-time phone calls, and whose wife often has to put dinner on hold. However, I get to know my patients well. As a result, they share many major events in their lives with me including the joys of birth, the sadness of death, and the shock of crisis. I can see their lives in a much more intimate way than any researcher or reporter can. My exam room is my research lab.

Early in my practice, one of the older doctors in the community died, and two others left town. They each had a large geriatric practice, and suddenly I was inundated with older patients. At first, my partners and I resisted and tried to maintain a "younger" practice. We even closed our practice temporarily to stop the influx of senior citizens. But after dealing with this special population, I discovered what a joy it was. I began to look forward to seeing my elderly patients and rapidly developed great respect and admiration for a number of them. I found them to be more compliant, more sincere, and more honest than some of my younger patients.

Age is no longer considered a matter of years but of function. Successful aging depends not only upon physical attributes, but also upon the relationship of the whole patient—body, mind and spirit. Because my practice contains an array of geriatric patients, I have studied extensively their medical needs and have attended multiple postgraduate conferences. Geriatric medicine is a newly expanding specialty, and much of the information in this book comes from new developments on the cutting edge of this field.

I thought about a title for this book for a long time. I wanted something that would truly describe the valuable people that I am writing about. Then one morning while in the shower, the title suddenly hit me. Vintage People! Vintage implies choice, value, being of a good period, representative of the best! It also suggests getting better with age. That is exactly what Vintage People do.

As with any profession, to become Vintage requires time. It takes maturity, experience and even failure. Many of the world's greatest accomplishments have come from Vintage People. When I graduated from medical school I thought I knew everything—but I was not a Vintage Physician. A good friend of mine is an airline pilot. He says it took years of flying experience to reach his current level of competency. The same holds true with life itself.

Our lives have seasons, just as nature has. To a certain extent, those seasons cannot be forced. We cannot hurry spring by reaching down and trying to pull the flowers from the ground. We cannot hurry summer by painting the cherries red. Nor can we hurry the bountiful harvest of fall. The vegetables, the fruits, and the grains cannot be rushed to maturity. Vintage wine takes time.

Vintage People also take time to mature and to learn about life. However, there may be a few shortcuts. We are not quite as dependent on the elements as are the seasons of nature. We have some control over our lives. We can watch the Vintage People around us and absorb those characteristics that make them Vintage. Some things we won't understand until we ourselves become Vintage. But as humans we can harvest some of the fruits of their growth, their mistakes, and their maturity. If you and I can incorporate what Vintage People have learned into our daily lives as we age, we too can be successful. There is *power* in aging! Vintage

People have discovered how to use that power to achieve what they want. Life really can get better as we age!

If we can arrive as Vintage People only a few years earlier than those around us, then we have those additional years to be filled with success, happiness and joy. We are allotted only a certain amount of time in this little ball of clay that we call our physical selves. Why not strive to spend as much of it as possible as Vintage People? Then we can begin to experience the abundant life that our Lord intended.

I trust this book will be an inspiration and motivation to Vintage People everywhere, empowering them to continue to achieve and to be successful—tapping into the power that comes with age. I envision the positive term "Vintage People" replacing the term "Senior Citizen" all over the world and becoming a household word! America's richest resource is truly our valuable Vintage People.

ONE

CHRONOLOGICALLY GIFTED

"To make a success of old age,
you have to start young!"
—Fred Astaire

I can't wait any longer! I'm going to have to re-schedule my appointment," an energetic eighty-two-year-old lady told my receptionist one morning when I was running late in seeing my patients. "I've got to get going! I have to deliver meals to some old people, who depend upon me."

My office staff related this story to me as I emerged from one of the examination rooms. They were still chuckling about this elderly lady's busy life and all the activities that she takes on. In our small Kansas town, my staff and I know most of the people that she volunteers to deliver meals to, and they are all chronologically much younger than she is. But this busy lady has been much more successful in aging than those younger individuals who are homebound, waiting for her to serve them.

I have been in family practice for over twenty years now, and it is said that as a doctor ages, his or her practice ages with them. As I began to see more and more geriatric patients, I became aware of dramatic variability in their health. Why was I seeing one sixty-seven-year-old for nursing home placement, and another ninety-two-year-old who was independent, living alone, and still driving her car? What causes one special group of older people to

1

remain motivated and creative, filled with self-confidence, hope, and spirituality?

Age itself doesn't seem to explain the difference. Perhaps it is just luck. But I don't think so. Early in my medical career, I strove to explain this difference on the basis of physical health and genetics but have found them to be less of a factor than most might imagine.

To learn the answer to this puzzle, I went right to the source—to successful older people in my practice, in my community, and across the nation. I asked them specifically what characteristics were responsible for their longevity and success in life. They trusted me and told me. I mailed out hundreds of letters asking them to respond in writing. Others I interviewed in person. For thousands I simply picked up bits of their philosophies and traits in the course of caring for their medical needs over the past two decades.

One of the major influences on my bedside manner and basic approach to patients came not from my medical school training, but from the teachings of Dr. Bernie Siegel, M.D. He is on the staff at Yale University and has published several books including *Love, Medicine and Miracles,* and *Peace, Love and Healing.* Dr. Siegel is best known for his work with cancer patients. Through his writing and lecturing, he has not only inspired and helped a number of cancer patients, but he continues to influence and to teach medical students, practicing physicians, and the medical profession as a whole.

The aspect of Dr. Siegel's work that has captured my attention and impressed me the most is his observation of a few exceptional patients. He was wise enough to notice that some of his cancer patients seemed to do much better than others, so he began to ask and seek out reasons why some patients respond in a superior way while others do not. This concept seems simple, but it shakes the very foundations of the medical profession.

Doctors have traditionally sought out pathology and disease. We did not study healthy people! Nor did we pay much attention to the non-scientific characteristics, beliefs, and attitudes that kept people out of our offices. There is a good reason for that. Historically, physicians only get paid for finding something wrong with the patient! Searching for the things patients are doing right to keep themselves healthy, and out of the doctor's office, doesn't pay very well!

Remembering Dr. Siegel's approach, I began to ask myself, "What are these healthy, alert, independent older people doing correctly that makes them this way?"

I stopped looking for what was wrong with these older folks and started looking for what was right with them. What are the characteristics they have discovered that make them so successful at aging? Are there secrets that we can learn to become even more successful as we age?

As I began to explore this concept, I discovered another amazing fact. Finding out what is right with someone is much easier than finding out what is wrong; it's easier than diagnosing a disease—because my patients would simply tell me! Every one of the exceptional older people I asked why they thought they were living so long and having such a healthy, successful life was eager to tell me. No one had ever asked them before, especially a physician. No X-rays or laboratory tests were required. Older patients were very willing to share their secrets of longevity and successful aging with me. They even told me they feel there is power in getting older!

Since I began questioning successful older people and listening to them, I have collected all kinds of opinions, beliefs, personal traits, characteristics, and philosophies about how to be successful as we age. Some are generic such as exercise and a good diet. Some are unique such as stretching and hanging from the top of a door frame several times a day. However, I began to notice immediately that a number of these characteristics fell into the middle of a bell-shaped curve and could help explain why these people do so well. A pattern emerges that we can all follow.

I heard a speaker once say, "That which is most personal is most universal." My patients have shared some of their most intimate and well thought-out ideas with me because I asked, listened, and took an interest in them.

Out of these ideas come some of the most valuable philosophies and information that we, as the younger generation, desperately need to hear. Vintage People have found how to be successful in life, just by living it and dealing with all the things that happen. From their experiences and maturity come a great number of valuable, new and refreshing philosophies that can benefit the rest of us as we age.

After collecting and studying these characteristics, I don't think that successfully reaching this stage of life is an accident. There may be some luck involved, but by learning what these people know we all have a better chance of aging successfully. I don't know at what point it happens, but even as grape juice somewhere along the line becomes valuable vintage wine, I believe that with the correct ingredients mixed effectively into the aging process, humans, too, can become valuable Vintage People.

Quantity of life versus quality of life

Today the chances that we can live to be one hundred years old and still be vibrant and healthy are better than ever before. We've witnessed a dramatic leap in life span in this century—from 47.3 years for the average American in 1900 to seventy-seven plus years today. The average American can expect to live about twice as long as their ancestors of just one hundred years ago. The "oldest old" (those eighty-five and above) make up the fastest-growing segment of our population. They have increased 232 percent between 1960 and 1990. And people over one hundred are increasing even faster!

The reasons are multiple. Better medical care and better public health measures are at the top of the list. Infant mortality, which for years skewed the statistics making the average life expectancy seem even lower, has improved dramatically. Nutrition is better and the environment safer now. Everyone still dies eventually; but now we have the chance of dying from heart disease, stroke, and cancer in old age, rather than from infectious diseases and childbirth in the early decades. Some clinical professors of geriatrics feel that we are simply beginning to fulfill our "natural biological heritage." However, no one knows for sure what that might be.

You may remember an article in *National Geographic* several years ago by a well-known scientist from Harvard University based on his interview of a man who was 186 years old in the area of Russia that is now Afghanistan. The scientist seemed to have discovered a "pocket of longevity" as there were many people over one hundred years of age living there. Excitement and speculation followed in scientific circles as to why these people lived so long.

Was it genetic, the goat milk in their diet, or some other factor? The excitement came to a screeching halt, when an exposition returned to study these people four years later—and found that everyone there had aged eleven more years! They used a different calendar; a different numbering system. There are no pockets of longevity!

How long can humans live if we are able to eliminate all pathology, diseases, and abuses from our bodies? Experts estimate anywhere from 70 years to 140 years! The one thing all reputable sources agree on is that the human body is not made to live forever. The Prophet Muhammadan says: "...there is one disease for which He has not created any remedy, which is old age."

I often discuss the "quality of life" versus the "quantity of life" with my patients. I definitely feel that quantity without quality is not desirable. It seems a mistake to add years to life without adding life to those years. It now appears that we may be able to have both! The image of people becoming sick and dependent as they age is no longer reality. We can keep our minds sharp and our bodies strong all our lives, even into the Vintage Years. Problems such as Alzheimer's disease, osteoporosis, or impotence are not part of natural aging. They are the result of disease, or pathology, not age.

Vintage People in my practice over eighty-five years of age are active, productive and healthy. Surprisingly, as the life-span in this country has increased, the disability rate has gone down. I once took care of a retired physical education instructor who lived to be 108. She remained alert and lived in her own home until the very end. This amazing lady had a "chin-up bar" secured to one of the doorways in her house. She did admit to me, however, that she had to give up doing chin-ups when she was eighty-eight!

More and more Vintage People are reaching the century mark. Most centenarians report that their nineties were essentially problem-free. The trick seems to be getting to the mid-eighties; if you make it that far, you'll be in a select group that are often more robust, and healthier, than people twenty years younger. The late, great George Burns understood this principle. He once quipped, "Once you get to be one hundred, you have made it. You almost never hear of anyone dying who is over one hundred!"

Making it this far seems to rule out all the people that were dealt "genetic lemons" in life. Certainly family history and genetics determines to some extent how long we will live, and what our morbidity will be. Unfortunately, many genetic disorders and familial diseases preclude longevity. The good news is that there are things which we can do to overcome such problems. Recently I met an eighty-one-year-old Vintage Lady named Doris, who gardens, travels, and is in charge of the Senior Citizens group at her church. When I asked her the secret to her successful life, her longevity, and her good health, she did not credit it all to her genes. Her mother and father both died in their early sixties. She had a brother who suffered with alcoholism and died in his early fifties. Rather, she stated, "I've always eaten right, don't drink or smoke, slept well, exercised and worked hard. I think I deserve credit for this!"

Perhaps she does deserve the credit. Research now shows that about seventy percent of the effects of aging may be due to factors that we can control. That is good news! Those factors are what we are going to discuss in this book. These are goals that we can all strive towards in order to improve our chances of reaching a tranquil stage of life and health that will let us become, what I am calling, one of the "Vintage People."

There is a giant difference between becoming an "old person" and becoming a "Vintage Person." The former has quantity of life only. The latter has quantity of life but has also discovered how to fill those years with quality of life. Vintage People are successful at life and have actually found power in aging. They are using it to their advantage. I like Art Linkletter's message for Vintage People: "If you're old, enjoy it!"

Experience

The most human of all traits is the ability to pass on information from one generation to the next. Isn't it wonderful that knowledge can be built upon over the years, decades, and centuries? Where would we be as a species if each generation had to rediscover fire? Instead, we have the unique ability to learn what an experience is like without actually having to go through the experience. I, for one, am glad I don't have to experience all the diseases my patients have in order to understand how to treat them successfully. Not to mention childbirth!

But there seems to be a built-in blockade to passing wisdom along successfully in one aspect of our lives. Everyone knows that we pass on physical information fairly well—scientific facts, discoveries about the world, and mathematical formulas, for example. But we do a horrible job when it comes to relaying information concerning relationships, philosophies of life, people skills, and moral values. In our youth we seem programmed to re-discover fire—and to get burned! Immaturity doesn't have the wisdom to listen. Walter Lippman in *A Preface to Morals* states, "It requires wisdom to understand wisdom; the music is nothing if the audience is deaf!"

There are just some things that each generation has to learn all over again for itself. Our parents watched us make mistakes in these interpersonal areas, and we will watch our children make the same mistakes. Perhaps it is because things of the heart take much more of a stimulus to make an impression on the brain. The heart seldom seeks wisdom. Take romantic love for example. We rarely pay attention to what others tell us. We forge ahead, often getting hurt until we learn some of the principles that someone could surely have taught us if we had just listened.

Other examples include such things as forgiveness, attitudes, the value of integrity, getting along with others and approaches to life. Each generation has to figure these things out for themselves. Some things just can't be taught. Norman Douglas describes it well: "Has any man ever obtained inner harmony by reading about the experiences of others? Not since the world began has it ever happened. Each man must go though the fire himself!"

But perhaps this is good. It's the way God planned it. Mankind has made great strides in the amount of information that is available, but almost no progress in relationships. We will trust the formulas of physics discovered by generations past when we prepare to build a bridge or a skyscraper. In the medical field we stake our lives on information from the past generations. But we won't believe our mother when she tells us to be home by midnight or we may get into trouble. Or will we believe the writings of the Bible telling us how to live successfully, without first wandering in the desert for forty years?

The main truth here is that we are going to make a lot of mistakes in our relationships with other people, and in our attitudes, and in our philosophies of life, on our way to becoming Vintage People. That is undoubtedly a vital part

9

of what makes us strong. As the popular saying goes, there must be enough shadows in our lives so that we can appreciate the sunshine. Experiences, especially the painful ones like death, lost loves, relationships, divorce, learning to control anger, and learning the consequences of holding a grudge, must be learned by all people if they are to become Vintage People.

There is an enormous wealth of information available from people that have been there—Vintage People who have learned from their mistakes so that we won't have to. They are the pilgrims who have discovered power in experience and maturity. The wise will listen!

The tranquil years

Much has been written about what is now called the "mid-life-crisis." In psychological terms, this is a period in life when one begins to re-evaluate where he is going. The classic example is the successful executive who has worked hard all his life to attain a certain goal only to find that this is not really the goal he wanted. He is busy climbing the corporate ladder only to discover in mid life that he has the ladder leaning against the wrong building! What he thought was so important when he was building his career may not seem nearly as important when he begins to realize that his children are slipping away, along with many other pleasures of life. All of the missed Little League games may begin to haunt him when he realizes those days are gone forever, but his work goes on endlessly.

In our current culture males seem especially vulnerable to this condition. However, as women become more and more career oriented, I suspect they, too, will be participants in this syndrome.

It seems that in mid life men become more emotionally sensitive, perhaps seeking the pleasures and fulfillment that they had sacrificed earlier in life.

Women, on the other hand, often find that their mothering, nurturing functions are no longer fulfilling, and they are looking for more independence. They are becoming more free, more intellectual, and more aggressive in seeking out what life has to offer. So, men and women are suddenly headed in opposite directions.

For both sexes, then, mid life often becomes a tortuous time when there are tremendous emotional changes taking place. This is a time of life when divorce is common. Career changes are common. Marital affairs arise. This is a time when a man may fall madly in love and marry a girl half his age. It's a time when job satisfaction is low, burnout is common, and clinical depression is frequent. During this time, it seems all the things previously worked for have lost their glitter. This is a time when men and women alike are asking, "Isn't there more to life?"

The positive side to all of this is that tremendous growth takes place during this period of our lives. Often, the partner that has "tolerated" an unfulfilled marriage will finally have the courage to correct it. People often become more "themselves" and begin for the first time in life to see what is really important to them. They may get out of a career they don't like. Or, they may discover that the career they are in can be extremely fulfilling if they just accept it. Disasters may happen, but on the other hand, this can signal the beginning of a fruitful and satisfying time in one's life.

In the ancient Tibetan Buddhist tradition of healing, significant times in a person's life are referred to as "Bardo." Bardo times are those periods which greatly influence an individual's life and are seen as times of tremendous personal growth. They include such times as graduation, beginning a new career, or religious enlightenment. Interestingly, the Tibetan Buddhist's life also includes the experience of illness, suffering, and loss as Bardo times. For Vintage People, aging is a Bardo experience—it may not always be a pleasant time, but out of it comes powerful inner growth.

I was discussing this concept with one of my older patients and she wrote me a beautiful comparison that made sense to me. I hope it will to you also:

> "I started life as a tender sapling in fertile soil. I was protected by the larger trees of the forest. Oh, I was vulnerable, and I was blown this way and that by the gusty winds of life, but nothing really bad happened to me. Finally, in mid life I found I had outgrown the protection of the other trees, but I was still soft and easily broken and twisted. Yet, during this stormy, emotional time of my life, I found myself becoming stronger—kind of like the gnarled old trees that survive on the windy, cold mountain slopes. Finally I discovered I had arrived at a very peaceful time in my life. Oh, the storms still come, but I am so much stronger now that not even the sharpest storm can interrupt the inner tranquillity that I feel!"

All of this to say that a more quiescent time is coming. The sun will shine again. There will be harmony again. Once the storms of change and gusty winds of insecurity are over in mid life, there is indeed a calm time in most people's lives. That doesn't mean that everything is suddenly perfect. Of course not! But the growth that has taken place seems to harden people. They are now tempered and much stronger than before. The new attitude and maturity they have gained during mid life, helps to usher in the tranquil years. I love the way Robert Browning, the well-known English poet, so eloquently describes this concept in his poem "Rabbi Ben Ezra"—

> Grow old along with me!
> The best is yet to be,
> The last of life, for which the first was made:
> Our times are in His hand
> Who saith, "A whole I planned,
> Youth shows but half; trust God: see all,
> nor be afraid!"

And so it is with Vintage People. They have passed through the turbulent mid-life years and finally reached calmer seas. This is the place of successful aging. This is the place where we would all like to be eventually. Of course, not everyone gets here, but those who desire to age successfully must recognize that they have control over how to get here. This is the noble goal—a goal certainly worth achieving. Vintage People realize there is power in maturity and wisdom. The book of Job sums it up by saying, "Wisdom is with the aged, and understanding in length of days." (Job 12:12)

Maturity

With the aging process comes a kind of magical state where things begin to change. Things begin to "fall into place." Vintage People begin to understand things that they either didn't notice or just didn't understand when they were younger. Maturity is a cycle—the more mature we become, the greater our propensity for maturity. Thus there is a snowball effect. Many of us roll around as a small clod for a long time before we begin to pick up snow. However, once we become a huge, heavy snowball, picking up more snow is easy. Herein lies the power of aging! Vintage People have the maturity to be wise. Age seems to be the price we humans pay for maturity.

I don't think we have a scientific explanation for this phenomenon, but we all know that it occurs. People have recognized it for centuries. The native Americans recognized it and bestowed honor upon their Vintage People for their wisdom. Oriental societies recognize the power of maturity and frequently place these individuals into areas of great leadership and teaching.

A great Jewish teacher and scholar described it in a letter that he wrote to his friends in Corinth: "When I was a child I thought as a child, I reasoned as a child. But now that I am an adult I have put away childish things." Because of their maturity—because they have put away childish things—Vintage People have more power than ever before in their lives for achieving the things in life that they really want, including happiness.

TWO

LIFE GETS BETTER

*"Youth is a gift of nature: Age is a
work of art."*
—Unknown

Lee Iacocca completely changed the course of Chrysler Corporation with his introduction of the "mini-van" at the age of sixty. Galileo published his last book at the age of seventy-four. Michelangelo, one of the most inspired creators in history, was appointed chief architect for St. Peter's Basilica at the age of seventy-one. After that, he went on to design the St. Peter's dome, which is his crowning achievement. That dome has stood as a symbol of authority in the western world over the centuries, including the model for our own national capital.

When he was eighty-five years old, Pablo Casals played a concert at the White House. He later published his "Reflections on Life" at the age of ninety-four. Susan B. Anthony resigned as president of the National American Women's Suffrage Association at age eighty but continued to be a regular speaker at their conventions until her death at age eighty-six. Bob Dole ran for president when he was seventy-two years old, John Glenn returned to space when he was seventy-seven, and Adolph Zukor was the chairperson at Paramount Pictures at ninety-one. At the age of ninety-six, George Bernard Shaw fractured his leg when he fell out of a tree that he was pruning!

Winston Churchill returned to the House of Commons as a member of Parliament at the age of eighty. When he was interviewed on his eighty-seventh birthday, a young reporter commented, "Sir Winston, I hope to wish you well on your one hundredth birthday." Churchill quickly replied, "You might do it. You look healthy!"

The list of great achievements by Vintage People goes on and on. But the point is this. Older is better! Researchers who studied the lives of four hundred famous and successful people discovered that thirty-five percent of the group's major accomplishments came between the ages of sixty and seventy. Twenty-three percent of their greatest achievements were done between the ages of seventy and eighty. Another eight percent didn't achieve their greatest contributions until they were past eighty! As one of my partners says, "it doesn't take a rocket scientist" to conclude that a majority of the world's greatest work has been done by Vintage People over the age of sixty.

We must not lose sight of this fact! Vintage People have unparalleled knowledge of the world and of what makes life meaningful. They are valuable. They possess experience; through experience comes wisdom; and wisdom is power. Vintage People use the power of their minds as a resource.

The ageless mind

Veterinarians look at a horse's teeth to tell the animal's age. Most people estimate another person's age based upon physical appearance, although that may be deceiving. Medically, there are a number of ways to determine the approximate age of the human body such as X-rays for bone age, and the appearance of degenerative effects like osteoarthritis. But no one has determined a way to specify age by looking at the mind.

The brain's capacity is almost inexhaustible. Our vision begins to fade at about ten years of age. Our hearing begins to decrease by about the age of twenty. By thirty our athletic abilities, muscular strength, and reaction time are all beginning to slow. But our mind is just beginning to work well! At fifty, our minds can be just as young as at twenty. At eighty we can be more productive mentally than we were at thirty because by that time we have gained something we didn't have earlier—experience!

Ever since I studied embryology in medical school, it has amazed me how two single cells coming together can form all the tissues of the human body. But the most amazing differentiation takes place in the cells that become the ten to twelve billion cells that form the human brain—a "three-pound power-house"—that makes us what we are. At a recent medical seminar, I heard the human brain compared to a computer—a computer made out of meat! But what an amazing computer! No man-made computer can even come close to the mysterious workings of the human mind. Even with all we do, the American anthropologist Margaret Mead estimates that only ten percent of our brain is ever used. Probably more like five percent for most of us. The potential is tremendous. Even if we lived ten times our current life span, our brains would still have more capacity to record information.

How does the brain do this? Neurophysiologists tell us that each cell has a set of microscopic tendrils that pass electrochemical messages from one cell to another. Without getting too technical, each of the ten billion or so nerve cells in the brain has between 1,000 and 6,000 connections to other cells. When all the possible connections are calculated, researchers estimate that there are roughly ten raised to the one-trillionth power combinations. (If you have forgotten your math, that's a pretty big number!) Every thought we have and every muscle we move is a result of thousands of these pathways firing. The truly amazing thing is that the more a person learns, the more connections are made. Switches are turned on and off in different combinations to record bits of information. As the brain is used, it becomes even more powerful! By the age of seventy, it is estimated that there are as many as fifteen trillion separate bits of information available to the average human mind.

This is where Vintage People begin to have an advantage. If the mind continues to be used, it becomes more and more effective. The memory banks are programmed with information that can be used in an ever-increasing number of potential combinations of thought. In this sense, an older brain is a better brain! It is a more powerful brain! The more tools we have at our disposal, the more creative we can be. No wonder so much has been accomplished by Vintage People!

I had a good friend in high school who became a carpenter. I watched him start his own business. At first he was limited in what he could build because of the tools that he could afford. He did small projects and re-invested much of his income into bigger and better tools. As he acquired more tools, he could do more, and bigger, projects. Eventually he had the gigantic cranes and heavy equipment to undertake the largest construction jobs. Building a skyscraper became easy once he had the right tools.

I think our minds work in this way. When a certain situation arises, Vintage People are able to reach in and take off the shelf the mental tool that is perfect for that project. The more tools, the greater the projects can become. Of course, the tools need to be maintained. The Vintage People I studied kept their brains sharp by putting new data in. Rather than spending time bemoaning the losses of aging, they seemed obsessed with the new things they were learning, the new skills they were acquiring, or the new project they were supporting. General Douglas MacArthur observed: "People grow old by deserting their ideals. Years may wrinkle your skin but to give up interest wrinkles the soul."

Vintage People enjoy keeping their minds active. Benjamin Franklin became a delegate to help draw up the Constitution of the United States when he was eighty-one years old. He could have elected to stay home in the rocking chair, or at his favorite fishing hole. But he chose to keep his mind sharp. At age eighty-four he addressed Congress about the abolition of slavery, a mentally challenging project that he was committed to supporting long before it became politically popular.

The human mind is ageless, but at any age it must be stimulated and used. An eighty-one-year-old patient of mine who still goes to work in his small store each day says he does it to keep his mind sharp, and that he will never retire. He explains it this way, "My doctor used to tell me I should retire and not work so hard. Of course, the doctor retired. He's dead now!"

The good old days

"If you want to experience the 'good old days,'" a retired physician told me, "throw away all your antibiotics, immunizations, medications, and sterile equipment in your office; and then sit around in the dark. And, oh yes! Don't forget to turn off the air-conditioner!" That's the response I got from most Vintage People when I brought up the subject of the "good old days."

A ninety-six-year-old Vintage Lady said, "The good old days? I'm not sure when that was! But I can tell you right now that I would rather live today than at any other time.

Now is the era men and women have dreamed about throughout history."

When I study the history of medicine, I agree with this lady. I wouldn't want to practice medicine at any other time in history. I'm not sure when the "good old days" were either. I sure don't find them in the history texts. I would not have wanted to be a physician in Bible times, when leprosy and infectious disease were rampant. Even aside from medicine, would we want to live in a political system where a ruler could decree that all male children in a certain province be killed—and it was done?

What if we only go back to the time when this country was settled? A third of the original settlers died that first year—but they still started Thanksgiving. Even before the discovery of penicillin, just a generation ago, life was tough. There is a record in one of my medical books of a family who lost all seven of their children, one each day, between Christmas and New Year's Day from diphtheria. One shot of penicillin could have saved all those lives. Early in my generation, there were huge hospital wards full of children who had been victims of polio—that doesn't happen any more.

The point is that we have it pretty good, and Vintage People realize it. Doug Larson says that "Nostalgia is a file that removes the rough edges from the good old days." People who honestly remember recall those rough edges. Will Rogers puts it a different way when he says, "Things ain't what they used to be and probably never was!" Memories are often more pleasant than the actual times.

One of the questions I asked the Vintage People I interviewed was, "Would you like to be twenty-one again?" I was greatly surprised at the answer they gave. Without exception they answered, "No!" The one stipulation that a number of the people wrote in was, "If I go back to age twenty-one, can I keep all the knowledge I've learned?" If the answer is no, then none of them want to be young again.

One eighty-four-year-old retired school teacher answered me like this: "If you would trade me my youth for my wisdom, the answer is overwhelmingly clear. I don't even need to think about it! I've struggled to learn what I have in life, and I'm very happy at my station in life. I have no desire to have to repeat the stages of my youth which I have already successfully survived!"

Vintage People like where they are and have a special place in society. Their generation has seen more changes than any generation that has ever lived. That experience and knowledge needs to be shared. Just think what they have seen. They have witnessed the creation of flight for the masses and watched America put a man on the moon. They have been eyewitnesses to the invention of television and computers. They have endured the devastation and losses of wars, and the great depression. They have sacrificed and done without. They have experienced death of friends, parents, spouses, and family members. They know life! Vintage People are important to our future. They have to be the advocates for disarmament, for using our rapidly growing technology for peaceful means, and for safe, renewable sources of energy. They have "been there—done that!" According to Vintage People, the good old days are now. Wake up America and listen to our most valuable resource—our Vintage People.

Age as a resource

A 65-year-old Vintage lady wrote me the following letter:

"I am tired of hearing about the glories of youth. It seems our culture associates positive things with being young: beauty, confidence, fun, and hope. On the other hand, everything negative is equated with being old, such as cynicism, fear, and helplessness.

I am no longer young and do not desire to be imma-
ture. At my age I know myself better, understand
more, and am more creative than at any other time in
my life. I have more self-confidence, more hope,
and more spirituality then I ever had in my youth. I
think that "old" is something positive!"

What a marvelous attitude! And there is so much truth
to what she said. This lady recognizes her maturity as a
resource for living successfully and enjoying life. I am
astounded when I think of the wealth of experience about
life, that Vintage People own. If you are in this group, you
have all the power within you to be successful as you age.
And each year should get better. Those of us not in that
group yet, can certainly learn about life and successful living from those who have forged the way.

Recently I had to seek out a physician for myself for an
ailment that I had developed—kidney stones. The idea of
wisdom and experience came in sharp focus. Did I want to
put myself in the hands of the young residents that I
instruct? Their scientific recall and knowledge of most
modern drugs and therapies is outstanding. In the final
analysis, I elected to choose a more experienced physician.
Why? Because I value his wisdom and experience over
knowledge. He has been there. He has seen this condition
hundreds of times before, but he realizes that each patient
is unique. The Vintage Physician learns to expect the
unexpected. He has learned, by "experience," what treatments work best in which patients. One of my instructors
once told me: "A prudent surgeon has the skill and wisdom
not to get into a situation where he needs his skill and wisdom!" That's the kind of doctor I want working on me!

The practice of medicine has changed dramatically over
the past quarter century, and so has our concept of aging. No
longer do older people retire to the rocking chair or their

favorite fishing spot. Nor is "old age" any longer synonymous with poor health and senility. Today, we are re-defining what is "old." In medicine we now view age as a matter of function, not years. If you are active, can feed yourself, dress yourself, and go to the bathroom by yourself, you are not old, even if you are one-hundred and three. If at age sixty you can't do some of those things, then you are old. A professor of geriatrics recently told me, "When you have seen one eighty-year-old patient—you have seen one eighty-year-old patient!" We are all unique individuals, regardless of chronological age.

Fortunately, we have now defined diseases such as Alzheimer's disease. And that is exactly what it is—a disease. It is not an expected result of normal aging. It is true that brain cells die as we age, but that starts the day we are born. Remember the huge capacity of the normal brain that we don't use? People are finding that if they stay active, both physically and mentally, they can continue to function very well into their eighth and ninth decades—and even beyond. "Normal" aging implies good health. All else is pathology.

As a nation we can harvest some of this rich insight from our healthy Vintage People. The greatest resource of this country has got to be its people. The American people have done more to change the world, in the shortest amount of time, than any other people in history. But I am afraid we are overlooking one of our most valuable resources. That is the wisdom, knowledge, and experience of our Vintage People. What a magnificent resource we have! Probably no other nation now has, nor has ever had, such a reserve of vibrant, active, healthy Vintage People. Think of the total years of experience we have to draw from in America today.

What does this mean to our nation? What does it mean to business, to social institutions, to schools and universities? What does it mean to government, to the use of our physical resources, and to medical care? And most of all, what does it mean to the rest of the country's population that has not yet reached that Vintage Age?

Private business, of course, is the first entity to begin to realize the potential of the Vintage Population. One only needs to look at all the "Senior Discounts" offered on everything from motel rooms, to movies, to restaurants, to new tires, to bank accounts. Businesses are not doing this out of benevolence for the older population on a fixed income. No, they are doing it because it is profitable! Vintage People are becoming a financially significant group, with political power as well. Again, if you are in this group, take advantage of your age. There are positive perks!

And what about the new trend about hiring retired persons to work as greeters at department stores, and in fast food restaurants, and at public parks? Again business is recognizing this great resource—because it saves them money! Vintage People often work cheaply and without benefits. They are extremely dependable and have the experience and wisdom to handle most any situation with style.

Yes, business is beginning to recognize this great resource, at least commercially. Many companies I have dealt with are relaxing their retirement policies. They are beginning to realize that perhaps older employees, in spite of being more costly because of seniority, are still very valuable to the company. Some corporations are elevating their Vintage People into consulting roles—the employee becomes part time, which saves the company money; but the company can still benefit from the employee's experience. Many professionals are also working longer. It is no longer unusual to see doctors, lawyers, barbers, pharmacists and small business owners maintaining their professions or businesses well into their seventies and beyond.

When I was a senior medical student, I had an attending physician as one of my instructors who had taught at the medical center for years—he had even written the book on physical diagnosis. But he also had a reputation for teaching through fear and intimidation. As a result, students avoided him as much as possible. One day, however, it was our turn, and he was making hospital rounds with four of us students and three residents. We all gathered around the bed of a certain patient, and he called on one of my fellow students to "present" the patient to him. The student did a fabulous job of relating the patient's past medical history and all of her symptoms. Then came the big question. "What is your diagnosis on this patient?" he asked the student.

We all held our breath. The student relied, "Sir, I think she has lupus." There was a collective sigh of relief as we thought the student had surely gotten it right and perhaps we were going to escape any grilling from this legendary instructor.

He peered over his reading glasses and said, "Very good! Now tell me why you think she has lupus."

The student thought carefully and began, "Well, sir, we did a set of blood chemistries on her and…"

Before he could even finish his sentence, the attending physician violently threw down the stack of medical charts he was holding and uttered a series of profanities! Everyone was shaking in his shoes, and we weren't exactly sure what had happened. Our instructor stood there as if in disgust and finally walked slowly over to the window. He leaned up against the window sill and let out a mournful sigh. After what seemed like hours, he finally turned to face the student who had answered. "Son," he said, "Come over here!"

Of course my fellow student went. The professor put his arm around his shoulder and escorted him to the window. "Look out here!" he told him. "Tell me what you see!"

"Well, sir," the student responded, "I see a tree!"

"Very good! What kind of tree is it?" the instructor asked.

"I think it is an elm tree, sir!" was the reply.

"That's right! Now, tell me how you know it's an elm tree."

"I guess just because it looks like an elm," was the student's petrified answer.

"That's right," the doctor replied. "You knew what kind of tree it was because you have seen one before. You didn't have to draw blood, or take any sap out of the tree to be tested, did you? The same thing applies to our patient here. She has lupus because it looks like lupus. I don't want to hear about blood tests; I want you to be able to identify a disease because you recognize it!"

What a traumatic experience! I have remembered the lesson well. This is the principle that comes with experience. Vintage People have the ability to immediately recognize situations, problems, and even relationship matters just by their appearance. No sophisticated analysis is needed. Perhaps their company doesn't need to spend thousands of dollars on market research or data gathering. Vintage People may be able just to look at the circumstances and know the answer. This also holds true for family matters, relationship problems, and the day-to-day dilemmas that present themselves in life. Here again, the resources of aging pay off.

By saying: "The next time I will..." or "From now on I'm going to..." it means that we are wiser today than we were yesterday. We cannot grow old without having our pathway scattered with storms, as well as with sunshine, with adversities, as well as joys, with heartache as well as laughter. But what tremendous wisdom can be gained along the way. And because of that wisdom, Vintage People have an inner power to be successful.

ACCEPTANCE

"God grant me the serenity to accept the things I
cannot change,
Courage to change the things I can,
and Wisdom to know the difference."

—Serenity Prayer

In studying Vintage People, I have found that the characteristics which make them successful fall into two categories. Some characteristics are cultivated. Vintage People
have worked hard to achieve these, and we will discuss
them later. However, along with maturity and longevity,
other characteristics are forced upon us. We have no control over them. These characteristics are a result of all the
incidents that "just happen" to all of us.

These inevitable events of life tend to make us stronger
and push us along our way to becoming Vintage People,
but seldom can we make them happen. They are totally random, circumstantial, and unpredictable. Some are heredi-
tary or genetic. Some are determined by the circumstances
of birth.

Occasionally, wise teachers and theologians have recognized this aspect of psychological growth and have tried
to help it along. Let me give an example. Our church helps
sponsor a retreat called "Camino." It has its modern begin-
nings in Spain, but originally mimicked certain Medieval

Monks who developed a very rigid program to help participants experience some of these maturing characteristics
that are usually random. I attended several years ago but
still remember the lesson it was teaching.

New participants are given very little information about
the retreat. They are driven to a church somewhere in
another city where they are to stay for three days. They are
left without a car and therefore cannot easily leave. Initia-
tion begins when all the watches and timepieces are gathered up so no one knows what time it is.

The first day, the recruits are awakened early in a loud
and rude manner. The food is bad—really bad. Green oat-
meal and unseasoned vegetables are served. The recruits
are given all kinds of ridiculous rules to remember and are
sent to the back of the food line if they don't perform properly. Not knowing the reasons for this uncomfortable situation, three other participants and I were planning our
escape to a McDonald's down the street.

The leaders had to keep reassuring us that there was a
reason for everything that was happening. Just "hang in
there," they kept reassuring us—"things will get better—
there is a reason for all of this!" We had to accept the things
that we could not change.

Close to the breaking point, when I had decided this
was all pretty stupid, and I was leaving anyway, things suddenly became wonderful! Gifts poured in from former participants. A wonderful banquet was served to us in a
beautifully decorated hall. We couldn't believe the transformation. We were suddenly in an atmosphere of love.

Then, it began to fall into place. We had been set up!
The whole thing—harassment, bad food, silly rules, and
lack of sleep—had all been done intentionally to simulate
the circumstances in the world that we cannot change.
These mishaps are just part of living in an imperfect world.

They have to be accepted. In this retreat we were being forced to accept the bad times so that the good times would be fully appreciated and savored. Once we were able to accept the things that could not be changed, our feast arrived, and we became Vintage Individuals—at least for this retreat.

We will all experience this on our way to becoming Vintage People. The world is going to make us conform to all kinds of ridiculous rules. Life is not fair! Bad things will happen, and there may be times when we want to escape. We will have to learn to tolerate and accept things that are beyond our control.

God didn't ask us if we wanted to be born male or female, black or white, American or non-American. As we age we will change, and our peers will change. Bad things will happen to us, and we won't always get our way. But somehow those that are going to become Vintage People recognize these factors in their lives, and finally arrive at a place where all these changes are accepted from life. Actually, Vintage People even go a step further. They begin to see these negative events as opportunities to grow. Then the abundant banquet of life really begins, and things get better than we ever expected them to be.

Circumstances of birth

Most of the Vintage People I interviewed were not born into circumstances that others would consider conducive to achieving success. As a matter of fact, most were born into poverty, by today's standards. Many had terrible family situations. Some were raised in a one-parent home. Some were physically abused as children. A number of them lost parents at an early age and had to learn to take care of themselves.

On the other hand, some have had supportive families. Some give credit to a nurturing family as the key to their success in becoming Vintage People. Others point to a specific role model—a parent, a relative or a family friend, who helped them on their way to achieving an understanding of life.

I was surprised to observe that race, color, sex, or physical handicaps do not have as great an effect as many might think. Remember here that I am talking about Vintage Status—people who are successful at life. I am not talking about earning large sums of money or about having big houses and cars. Instead, I am talking about a human quality that can be achieved with or without material success. Unfortunately, if you are black, statistics in this country show that, on an average, you may earn less money. Statistics also show that if you are female, you may earn less money; and if you have a handicap, you may not get as large a share of material wealth. But that does not mean that you cannot be a successful person with life experiences to share with others. In fact, anything that presents a challenge in life may actually make Vintage Status a little easier. Many Vintage People have not only overcome their handicaps and social injustices but have actually used those circumstances to grow creatively.

One of the most interesting gentlemen that I have been privileged to care for in my medical practice was an American Indian. He died when he was ninety-nine. Up to that time he remained active and very alert. He had an advantage over the general population because in his culture, age and wisdom were seen as synonymous. The hardships and discrimination that he described while growing up are hard for many of us even to imagine. Yet he was not angry. I will never forget a statement he made to me one day when I was preparing to do a minor procedure on him. I commented that it might be somewhat uncomfortable for awhile. He replied, "All the pain that I have endured in my life makes me what I am today—hard as granite, sly as a fox, and as wise as the wisest Indian Chief who ever walked this land! And I would not exchange it for the easy life!"

The point is that most successful Vintage People living today have not led a charmed life. They were not born into ideal circumstances. And surprisingly, I found this to be universally true. It is known that approximately seventy-five percent of the world's leaders were born into poverty, had a major handicap to overcome, or were abused as children in some way. The circumstance of birth does not totally determine what we are going to make of our lives. You and I alike can become Vintage People no matter what our birth status has been. Paradoxically, the things that seem to be disadvantages may in the long run end up making us strong!

Diversity

I remember one of my professors in medical school talking about how we all become more diverse organisms as we age. Of course, he was talking about physical diversity. As we get older, we are prone to an increasing number of pathological conditions. Older people have a wider variety of diseases. About ninety-five percent of the diseases in newborns involve either congenital abnormalities or the respiratory system. At the other end of life, older people may suffer from thousands of different afflictions. I have shelves of medical texts trying to describe these ailments, from several hundred types of cancers, to diabetes, to kidney failure, to TB, to AIDS, to thousands of conditions so rare that they remain a medical oddity. It has always seemed to me that God could have chosen about ten diseases for humanity to die from. That would have been enough! Why do we need people to die from such things as cancer of the fingernail or die like the patient that developed blood poisoning after he cut himself shaving? Our life-styles, occupations, environmental exposures, and waning immune system may play a part. One thing is certain: as we age we become much more of a physically diverse group. We age at very different rates.

But as we age we also become much more divergent in our personalities and our psychological makeup. Infants come into this world with only a set of programmed instincts to follow. I'm not trying to insinuate that infants are simple beings, because research has shown us that infants are already extremely complex creatures at the time of birth. Nor am I implying that genetics and family history have very little to do with our future behavior and personality. What I am saying is that as human beings go, we are the most alike when we are born than we will ever be again.

Infants in the nursery will look more alike, act more alike, and respond more alike than any group of humans ever will again during their lifetimes. Watch children at play. A group of three-year-olds will respond in a fairly predictable way. First graders begin to be a little more diffuse. I recall that in the first grade I pretty much felt that all six-year-olds would respond the same as I would. By junior high, I began to notice a few kids that were different. Their behaviors were different, and their life-styles began to be different from mine. By the time I started college, I began to wonder if anyone, except me, was "normal." Yet even through medical school, with a multitude of diverse personalities, there was still some feeling of collegiality. Perhaps our schools foster that. After all, everyone who receives a certain degree is expected to have met certain standards. Colleges strive for a certain sameness or "product mold."

However, once out in the real world, every human develops at his own rate, and through all the life experiences that come his way. Our subconscious brain records all the good and bad experiences we have each day. And just like the computer, if we put garbage in, we will get garbage out. If we put positive images in, we will tend to think in positive and hopeful terms. But our thoughts remain individual.

Imagine what diverse input I may have experiencing the things I see as a medical doctor, versus what a politician, or cab driver, or a sports star may see. Our experiences in life are going to determine our thought process and how we view things. Medical school has changed me forever! The first time I saw a baby born or watched a beating human heart in surgery, I was changed. I remember dissecting a cadaver and developing an appreciation for the human body. I have had the unique privilege of sharing in my patients' deep secrets and in times of tragedy and death. Having experienced all these things makes me different—more diverse—than my elementary school friends who went into other careers. After having been a doctor, or a teacher, or a mechanic, or a computer programmer, or a policeman, for thirty years, we are going to be much more diverse than we were in the first grade!

But this is good! We couldn't accomplish much in the first grade. It may be harder to strike up a technical conversation as we become more diverse, but look at all the wisdom and knowledge that has been gained if we will share it. I have a good friend who repairs television sets. We often tease each other about our technical knowledge. But we both know that I would have about the same amount of luck repairing a television set as he would have removing an appendix! But together we can use our skills to each other's advantage.

This is one of the characteristics of becoming a Vintage Person over which we have very little control—we can control ourselves, but not the diversity of others. As we successfully move toward that type of maturity and human wisdom, a great deal of diversity is going to develop and continue to increase. Vintage People use this to their advantage. Diversity fosters a lot of "weird" beliefs, and a lot of ideas that are different from our own. But just when we need it most, God seems to give Vintage People more tolerance for those that are different from them as well.

Hardening

A number of years ago a very wise gardener taught me how to start tomato plants indoors. I had done this a number of times before, but often when I set my nice succulent plants outdoor in the garden, the wind broke them off, the rain pounded them into the mud, or the hot sun caused them to wilt. At any rate, they were not what you would call "successful" tomato plants. And yet I had raised them so carefully, providing them with plenty of fertilizer, light, and moisture. They looked beautiful and green, without a blemish. But they could not survive the harshness of suddenly being transplanted outdoors.

Later I learned from the wise gardener that I had not "hardened" my plants. Their lives had been so pampered and sheltered that they could not even survive the consequences of nature out in the vegetable garden. I learned that the plants did much better if I slowly began to prepare them by occasionally withholding water, setting them outside on sunny days, and letting the heat and wind wilt their leaves for gradually increased periods of time. Often the beautiful succulent leaves were torn, and had browned edges, but those plants were tough and would survive.

This parallels life in so many ways. Until I was about forty years old, I was very much like the tender, friable young tomato plant, that had never really faced adversity. I had not been hardened. But all that changed with a divorce, the accidental death of my oldest son, and a couple of other failed relationships. God was hardening me, and doing a very effective job of it!

As Mother Theresa said, "I believe that God will not give us a burden greater than we can bear. But I just wish He didn't trust me so much!" One Vintage Lady stated it this way: "There are some things in life you don't ever get over. You just accept it and go on the best you can."

This hardening is a characteristic that is strong in all the successful Vintage People I have ever encountered. It seems to be paramount. Most of the successful older people in the world today have experienced tremendous losses, gigantic setbacks, and heartbreaking emotional and physical pains.

The pattern that has emerged from the older people I have studied is that their "hardening" often began very early in life. As mentioned earlier, most were born into poverty. They struggled through the great depression and often went without material things. They saw atrocities of war and lived with the threat of war most of their lives. By the time they reached retirement age all had experienced the death of a close friend, and many had lost a sibling, a spouse, or a child. Of course most had experienced the loss of parents. Yet, there seems to be a positive side to this hardening—creating a more successful human being.

Hardening also follows the physical side of aging. Medically, it is a known fact that as we age we become hardened as far as pain is concerned. Diagnosis can be difficult in older patients because of the endurance nature tends to give us as we age. Older people seldom have headaches or migraines. Likewise, older people with pneumonia, acute appendicitis, kidney stones, and gall bladder attacks may complain very little of discomfort.

I have even seen people over the age of seventy-five suffer a major heart attack and have absolutely no chest pain. All of these conditions would totally flatten younger individuals that have not been hardened. Maybe this comes as a result of the pains we endure in life, or perhaps it is a favor of nature to prepare us for the tougher times that come with aging. But it is nevertheless true.

Just like the tomato plants, adversity and stress can make us stronger. But this is where the similarity ends. Tomato plants have very little choice as to how they respond. As humans we have a very definite choice as to how we react. Adversity can stimulate us to grow and to become much stronger persons, or it can drive us into pity and pessimism. Successful older individuals have somehow allowed the former to happen. Let us look at the characteristics that allow this to happen.

A man I will call Guy has taught me this valuable lesson. He continually serves others by delivering "meals on wheels," driving the elderly (some of whom are younger than himself) to the doctor's office, and even leading a Sunday School class. He is always upbeat and happy. No one can experience his presence for more than a few minutes without feeling better!

But Guy has not had a charmed life. He lost his wife after a long illness, and has had major health problems of his own. He has had financial worries, and others have taken advantage of his generosity on several occasions. He grew up in a poor family and never achieved the material rewards that he would have liked in life. Yet he has turned this adversity into a blessing.

Think about that paradox! How can life get someone down who takes bad things and turns them into blessings?

This is somewhat akin to the apparent frustration of the ancient Roman rulers in the early Christian era. The Christians were a group who perceived persecution as a blessing. What could be done to these people? Persecuting them only made them stronger! Vintage People who have been successful in life, have learned this skill. When life deals them a blow, they just come back revitalized and stronger than ever.

Another eighty-two-year-old lady I have treated for years has just completed chemotherapy for leukemia. Prior to that her husband died from cancer. Several years ago her house burned to the ground, and she lost all of her possessions, including family heirlooms, pictures, and other objects of sentimental value. Because of her impaired immune system, she frequently develops skin cancers that grow rapidly and need to be removed.

I was removing a large skin cancer from her arm one afternoon, when in the course of conversation she commented how lucky she was. My nurse asked, "How can you consider yourself so lucky when you have had so many bad things happen?"

"Oh," she replied, "I've had a lot of things happen that I didn't like at the time. But they happened anyway! I am very lucky. If I hadn't gotten leukemia I would have never known how many people care and love me. Every time tragedy touched my life, I was determined to take it and make something good happen! It's not easy, but I've done it!" This lady realized that adversity is unavoidable. So why not use it to strengthen ourselves? Albert Einstein suggested that "in the middle of every difficulty lies opportunity."

It is amazing when we look at history how many great people have used adversity to grow and to create opportunity. Abraham Lincoln lost far more elections than he ever won. Beethoven went deaf—the most tragic thing that could happen to a musician, but he still completed some of his most beautiful works after that. The Apostle Paul wrote many of his renowned epistles while confined to a prison cell awaiting, as far as he knew, execution. The Greek orator Demosthenes overcame a lifetime of stuttering to rally people with his touching speeches. Helen Keller, who was deaf and blind from early childhood achieved a greatness that few have ever reached. She stated, "The marvelous richness of human experience would lose something of rewarding joy if there were not limitations to overcome. The hilltop hour would not be half so wonderful if there were no dark valleys to traverse."

But does that mean we should welcome adversity into our lives? Should we go out of our way to have bad things happen? No, I don't think that is human nature. We all try to avoid tragedy if at all possible. There is a bit of a paradox here. Just as one cannot "plan" for "spontaneity," true tragedy cannot be invited into our lives. The truth is that most of the really bad things that happen to you and me are things that we have no control over. If we could control them, they won't happen.

Of course, at times we unknowingly set ourselves up for disaster. Driving after drinking alcohol, for example. Every weekend when I work in the emergency room, I see victim after victim of alcohol-related accidents. Such behavior is indeed asking for tragedy in one's life. The disastrous outcomes often seem to surprise the people involved more than they surprise me. These people didn't think it would happen to them!

I'm sure you can think of many other examples where people seem to be asking for trouble. But when you talk to such people, they don't seem to be engaging in this behavior on purpose. They are not consciously willing tragedy upon themselves. Some psychologists would argue that such people have self-destructive tendencies because of underlying subconscious problems, but when I talk to them in the emergency room, I sense that they would still avoid the adverse outcomes if they could.

Successful Vintage People realize that we live in an imperfect world where tragedy strikes, wars occur, people die, and we are sometimes disappointed in our fellow human beings. Enough bad things are going to happen that we don't need to set ourselves up for them. I think the opposite is true. It is our job to avoid pitfalls, but be willing to accept them. Psychologically this is healthy—kind of a win-win situation. If good things are happening, we confirm the blessings we are being given. If bad things happen, we can rejoice that something good will also come of that.

I heard a speaker say that if you interviewed people one year after they had won the lottery, ninety-five percent would be unhappy, saying that the lottery had wrecked their lives. According to this speaker, if you went to the home of a disciple of Carl Jung, the great Swiss psychiatrist, and said, "I have just won the lottery," he would say, "That's too bad, but if we work hard maybe we can get you through this without too many catastrophes!" If you went to this same person and said, "My house just burned down and I've lost all that I have," they would say, following Jung's teachings in psychology, "Great, let's open some wine and celebrate—something good will come of this!"

James, the brother of Jesus, wrote to the early Christians: "When all kinds of trials crowd into your lives, my brothers, don't resent them as intruders, but welcome them as friends! Realize that they have come to test your endurance. But let the process go on until that endurance is fully developed, and you will find you have become men (and women) of mature character...." (James 1:2-4, J. B. Phillips edition).

With this attitude we can be successful in life, particularly in the upper decades when adversities seem to be increasing in frequency and severity. When we reach this point, depression, resentment, anger and stress will no longer have a grip on how we perceive and live our lives. I'm told that the ancient Chinese symbol for "crisis" has a dual meaning: danger and opportunity.

Consider the words of an anonymous poet:

Looking back, it seems to me
All the grief, which had to be,
Left me when the pain was o'er
Richer than I'd been before.

Adolescence of retirement

A medical cartoon in one of my examination rooms shows an old man sitting in the doctor's waiting room with his cane. The young receptionist sitting at a desk nearby is filing her nails and looking bored. The old man shakes his head and says, "Youth is wasted on the young." The young receptionist looks up from her boredom and replies, "Retirement is wasted on the old!" Stated another way, a Bulgarian proverb says: "There would be miracles if youth could know and age could do."

In a way, aging, and especially retirement, is a lot like adolescence. Both periods of time happen whether we want them to or not. There is no control. Both involve a time of tremendous change in one's life. In both, the body is changing and we have to learn to make adjustments for it, but in opposite ways. While adolescents are getting used to the rush of hormones, older people are adjusting to menopause and reduced hormone production. Adolescents are experiencing increased hair growth, while older people watch their hair come out in the sink! The pimples of adolescents have given away to wrinkles and age spots. Both groups spend a fortune on complexion medications!

These two groups have a lot of psychological similarities as well. They are both making adjustments to live in their new world. They are learning new social skills. The ways in which other people relate to them are changing. Society's expectations are suddenly becoming different. Good or bad, people begin to stereotype both groups.

Just as in adolescence, when we grow older we have to decide what we want to be. What role are we going to play now? What comes after retirement? Adolescents actually spend a lot more time preparing for their function in society than do most retiring persons.

I went to school and trained for twenty-three years before I "grew up" and began my medical practice. I suspect when I retire I will have just some vague notions about doing volunteer work and traveling. Not much more planning than that!

As we approach retirement we certainly have a lot more experience and a lot more wisdom to make these decisions than do adolescents, but we seldom apply those skills. The reason is probably that neither the adolescent nor the aging adult knows with certainty what they are headed for. Milan Kundera states it this way: "We leave childhood without knowing what youth is; we marry without knowing what it is to be married; and even when we enter old age, we don't know what it is we're heading for: the old are innocent children of their old age. In that sense, man's world is the planet of inexperience."

Would we want it any other way? Just as adolescence is a challenging and exciting time of life full of possibilities, the Vintage Years of life can be as well. However, it is good to prepare, to have a plan and goals.

Most of us spend our working life planning financially for our retirement—the government even thinks it so important that they will do it for us should we fail to! But many of us do not spend any time at all preparing emotionally and socially.

Just as the behavior of adolescents is often hard to understand, there are a few things I don't yet understand about some of the Vintage People I have known. Two Vintage People I know retired recently. One was a physician in my group, and another was a retailer who owned and operated a pharmacy. Both worked into their late seventies, and both continue to be active in the community.

When they retired, their colleagues, patients and customers wanted to pay tribute to them. However, both refused any attention and even refused to allow the local paper to do an article about them. Neither wanted any type of reception. Both had to be coerced into at least coming to a farewell dinner put on by their employees and co-workers. Many people truly wanted to return something to these Vintage Men for the care and respect they had shown towards their patients and customers throughout the years.

In typical teen-age fashion, neither of these gentlemen could give me a good answer as to their hesitancy in accepting any public praise other than they didn't want to. Neither did they wish to talk about it. I'm not sure they understood either. I arrived at two conclusions. First of all, perhaps they were embarrassed or felt a little guilty that they were "giving up." Secondly, I think they might view any public display as "the end." Kind of like a "career funeral." Perhaps any public recognition would be too emotionally taxing or emotionally charged. And, of course, there may be other factors that I don't understand yet.

This behavior could be just another characteristic of Vintage People. They may view retirement as merely another change in their life, like a promotion, or renewing their medical license for another year. Perhaps for the physician it was viewed as I would view attending a medical seminar—just another accomplishment. Whatever the reasons, I know both of these gentlemen well enough to know that this will not be the end for either of them. Like all Vintage People, they will both continue to contribute to life in a number of ways.

George Bernard Shaw reflects on retirement as a Vintage Person when he writes: "Life is no brief candle to me, it's sort of a splendid torch which I've got to hold up for the moment, and I want to make it burn as brightly as possible before handing it on to future generations. I personally don't believe in retiring. I believe we should live our lives in crescendo; that we should continue to make significant contributions in whole new ways all the way through our life. We may retire from a job or from an occupation, but we always retire to extremely meaningful projects."

FOUR

KNOW THYSELF

"The unexamined life is not worth living."

—Plato

A number of years ago I read a cartoon in the "Peanuts" column by Charles M. Schulz. It went something like this: Lucy approaches Charlie Brown and asks, "Charlie Brown, do you know what's wrong with you?"

Charlie Brown answers emphatically, "No," and walks off.

True to her nature, Lucy shouts after him, "What's wrong with you, Charlie Brown, is that you don't want to know what's wrong with you!"

Charlie Brown doesn't qualify to be a Vintage Person! One of the chief characteristics that came up repeatedly in the Vintage People I interviewed was their ability to evaluate themselves—to know themselves. They are aware of their abilities, their goals, and their emotions. Vintage People tend to use self-awareness to their advantage in all they do.

A retired theology professor on my hospital's board of trustees stated it like this: "I think it is important to know yourself as well as you can. By that, I mean be aware of the parameters or limits of possibility that you are capable of pursuing. As a person grows older, he or she loses some of the energy that was once there. Recognizing this enables the person to work with what they have to the fullest extent. It is surprising what you can do if you do not over-extend yourself but be careful about what you can do. I suppose to sum up all of this the most important thing is to follow the maxim of the oracle of Delphi: 'Know thyself!'"

There is tremendous wisdom in those words.

Recognition

Vintage People feel that "knowing themselves" is para-mount to successful living as they age. By that, I mean an awareness of their parameters or abilities, realistically in tune with their changing stages of life. Our position in life changes constantly, and we need to know where we stand. Vintage People have discovered how to evaluate them-selves in proper perspective, but in addition to recognize their limitations as well as their assets. Self evaluation is an extremely valuable ability at any juncture of life, but one that Vintage People seem to capture early on.

An uncle of mine, whom I consider a Vintage Person, has had a rags-to-riches type of life. In spite of a polio handicap and no formal education following high school, he tends to be successful at everything he tries. Starting as a mechanic working on airplanes, he worked his way into an executive position for a major airline by the time he retired. Even after retirement he has continued to be busy on advisory boards and even helped restore and rebuild an antique airliner—and has helped fly it to air shows. He recently built and is operating his own airport!

He explains how "knowing himself" has created his success: "As president of a 4-H club for three years, while in school, I learned leadership and to accept responsibility; also that people believed and trusted me. I discovered that learning seemed to come rather easy for me and I took advantage of it."

He began to evaluate himself early in life. He was able to discover his talents and how to then use them for his own success. Some people learn this later in life than others, but it is never too late. We are all given talents, the Bible assures us of that. It is up to us to discover what they are. However, in unfolding these discoveries, age has the benefit of experience, and youth is at a disadvantage. As we age we will have tried more things. At some things we will have succeeded, and at some we will have failed. But as we gain experience we should examine ourselves and notice what works for us. The more endeavors we have tried, the easier it should become to "Know Thyself."

Vintage People have developed a method to recognize their assets and to evaluate themselves in proper perspective. This is an ongoing process for all of us! Let's explore what works.

Pace yourself

A good doctor recognizes his or her limitations. In the medical profession, I have a great deal of respect for the physician or other health care worker who says, "I don't know" and seeks consultation when confronted with a difficult diagnosis or treatment. Likewise, I was very impressed when many of the Vintage People in my interviews related to this principle when they simply stated, "I know I am old." Rather than trying to remain young, or deny their age, they recognize the toll of aging as a stage of life. They don't fight it; they take advantage of it. They realize that what they have lost in physical agility and mental quickness they can make up in experience and depth of wisdom. They pace themselves and recognize their limitations.

My own father put it this way: "Avoid stress. Know when to say No. Don't take on more than you can do well." He illustrated his point by describing a sixty-five-year-old woman at his church who couldn't say No. She apparently felt obligated to take on more and more projects—then didn't do any of them well. She was always under criticism for failing to complete her projects or doing them poorly. She was not considered a Vintage Person but was viewed as old, forgetful, and somewhat incompetent. In reality, none of these perceptions were true, but they came from a lack of pacing herself and doing just those things that she could do well. Successful Vintage People have learned what their limitations are and what they are good at accomplishing.

I am sometimes asked to perform physical examinations to recommend older people for driver's license renewal in Kansas. I'm always torn in my decisions. If I deny a driver's license to one of my patients, I am taking away his total independence and handing him a sentence to be homebound. On the other hand, if I recommend him for his license, I may be putting that person, as well as society as a whole, in danger. What if the person runs into a school bus?

I must admit that I have found some consolation in statistics showing that older people are less likely to be aggressive drivers and are not the menace to society they sometimes appear to be. While older drivers have the highest crash rate per miles driven of drivers in all age groups, they drive the least number of miles. Consequently, they account for the least number of fatal accidents, and they have the lowest crash rate per licensed driver of all age groups.

Most accidents involving older drivers are of the fender-bender variety. And here is why. When I question these people about their driving, they recognize their limitations. They pace themselves. They tell me they wait until rush hour traffic is over to go out. They almost never drive at night. They drive slowly. They map out their route and take streets that are less traveled to reach their destinations. They concentrate on their driving because they recognize their decreased reflexes, decreased visual acuity, decreased hearing, and other physical limitations may place them at a greater risk of being involved in an accident.

Compare this to the younger drivers who feel they are invincible. They turn the stereo up, experiment with excessive speed and do a number of other functions while attempting to drive a car. They take risks relying upon their alertness and quick reflexes to protect them. They weave in and out of traffic, tailgate, and even challenge other drivers in an aggressive way. Who is safer on the street? To my way of thinking, experience and wisdom always win over unnecessary risks and quick reflexes. I must admit that these days when I get on an airliner, I feel reassured when I see a little gray in the pilot's hair!

This principle can be demonstrated further with an example of two physicians I have worked with over the years. They both were tremendous surgeons in their time and saved many lives in our community. However, as they aged the first surgeon didn't recognize his limitations. He didn't learn to pace himself. He continued to practice just as he had always done. However, at a certain point, our medical review committee began to notice that his dexterity wasn't the same. His cases took longer to perform. Next, we noticed that his judgment was not as sound as it had been in his younger days. His operative complication list began to grow. He explained all of this by saying that the patients he had to work on were more ill than earlier ones. Meanwhile, patients remembered him as he had been many years ago and still trusted him completely. But more and more of his patients had to be taken back to surgery for bleeding or other complications. Sadly, he didn't seem to recognize any problem.

As members of the medical staff, we saw his performance dropping below the acceptable standard and were obligated to step in before anyone was seriously injured. He fought our actions vigorously and felt the younger doctors were just trying to steal his patients. He had missed this characteristic of becoming a Vintage Person—recognizing one's limitations. He had not learned his "limits of possibility." He was fighting the aging process rather than adapting to it. There were still enormous areas in the medical field where he could have performed well and continued to be valuable to his patients if he had paced himself and recognized his limitations. He was a frustrated and unhappy physician at a time when he should have been enjoying life as a Vintage Person.

Contrast this first physician with another surgeon in town. He was still a competent surgeon at the age of seventy-two, when he examined himself and felt it was time for him to give up the surgical part of his practice. There was no battle with the medical staff as he was still very competent. As a matter of fact, most of us tried to talk him out of this move as we thought it premature. But he stuck to his decision and began an office practice with regular hours and two days off a week. He recognized that he needed more rest. He was always available for a surgical opinion or consultation with any of us, and we frequently relied upon his experience and wisdom to help us with difficult cases. But he never again picked up the scalpel. Over the years he decreased his practice slowly and just recently retired totally at the age of seventy-seven. Now he is running a travel agency which had always been a dream of his.

Now I ask you, which of these two qualify as a Vintage Doctor? Which one was truly successful in his aging process?

This is a good story, you may say, but haven't you been encouraging older people to continue working? Isn't work itself a sign of a Vintage Person? Many who work past retirement age are very successful, not only in their health, but also in their lives. One of the most frequently given secrets of longevity and prosperity from my interviews with Vintage People was "hard work!" So, how do we know when to stop, when to give up something, when to admit defeat?

First of all, I don't think acknowledging our limitations is defeat. Knowing oneself and pacing oneself are positive accomplishments. Thoroughly examining oneself requires wisdom. It requires contemplation, judgment, and conscientiousness. Perhaps it involves one's spiritual side. Perhaps it requires talking it over with God, or even leaving it in God's hands.

Whatever the answer, I'm sure that each one will be as individual as each Vintage Person on earth. Everyone has to decide what is right for him or her. Vintage People tend to have the wisdom, experience, and judgment to make that determination successfully.

Journaling

The history of modern man is a written history. From classical times on, man discovered that there is something enduring, something magical about writing things down. A written piece helps the human mind remember and makes what is written seem more real than what is spoken. It can "soak in" better. It can be repeated, and it never changes.

Emmitt Smith, who played for the Dallas Cowboys, won three Super Bowls and four rushing titles. One time during an interview a reporter asked him his secret to playing so successfully. Smith attributed his accomplishments to writing a list of goals at the beginning of each season. He explained that when he was a student at Escambia High in Pensacola, Florida, his football coach used to say, "It's a dream until you write it down. Then it's a goal." Smith branded those words on his heart and has continued to make lists and goals on and off of the football field. Writing it down has made the difference.

Other successful people have followed this principle as well. According to his *Autobiography,* Benjamin Franklin put into writing a series of resolutions which he attempted to follow as a young man. Some were difficult, such as Resolution Number 2: "Silence—Avoid trifling conversation." Resolution Number 3 was: "Order—Let all your things have their places." And the most ambitious one of all was Resolution Number 13: "Imitate Jesus and Socrates!" Ben kept these resolutions written in a small book and reviewed them each day. At the end of the day he would judge his performance and place a small check mark by each one that he had broken.

My point here concerns writing things down or "journaling." Most of the Vintage People I have talked to have learned that making personal, written records is well worth the effort. Most great historical figures kept diaries or journals. Contracts are always in writing. Businesses put their mission statements in writing. A man and a woman can live together, but look what a difference that little written marriage license can make! God wrote down the tablets he gave to Moses. The Bible is written word. Letters carry more of an impact than a phone call. Things that are written are perceived by the human mind as being more important than those that are only spoken. We write down things such as grocery lists and the paper boy's address. Aren't the goals and directions of our lives at least as important?

One of the Vintage People who responded to my request for information sent me a list of well-thought-out points. I could tell that he had spent a large amount of time working on his response. He closed his letter with these words: "Thanks for the opportunity to write these things down. I probably have not been much help to you, but it was good for me."

If you have never tried writing things down, you really should. I suggest it to my patients all the time. It can be as simple as recording a number from one through ten on the calendar each day to indicate how you felt that day. Following this method may show a pattern that can help diagnose such things as migraine headaches, PMS, or depression. A diary can be used in this way, or you can have an elaborate list of goals on the computer. But make your list truthful and personal—it's just for you to see. If it doesn't reflect your genuine feelings, then it won't be helpful.

It is even better if you can carry a small notebook, like Benjamin Franklin. Jot down those fleeting mental breakthroughs and "openings" that come your way during the day. You can think on those later. If you are like me, your mind may be dealing with so many things during the day that by the end, you remember only the major happenings. I have found that many important thoughts and ideas sneak into my mind and out again without fanfare. Catch them while they are there, or they may be gone. Once they are written, they have been captured.

Vintage People tell me it is important to snag a brilliant idea while it is there, but it is even more important to write down your goals and your philosophy of life—kind of a personal "Mission Statement," if you will. All major corporations, businesses, churches, and organizations have a mission statement. Why shouldn't each of us have one for our life? Motivational courses often recommend that we stand in front of a mirror and repeat our mission statement in a positive way. Sounds silly at first, but it does work! People feel better about themselves.

About half of the Vintage People I know have a written statement they use to keep themselves on track. They suggest we all do it. It doesn't need to be long and can be in our own language. Many Vintage People say they find this helpful, especially when they get mired down in the details of life. They can stop, review their written declaration and remember what is really important to them. One eighty-eight-year-old lady who is a retired pharmacist told me that her mission statement contains the phrase, "keep a cheerful attitude." Another phrase is "count your blessings." "That statement always reminds me that when someone asks 'how are you?' that is my trigger to quickly count all of my blessings. I don't take a lot of time to recount all my ailments and troubles—they don't want to hear them anyway!"

A common time for Vintage People to put their goals into writing is at the time of their retirement. Of course these can change and can be amended at any time, but research has shown that if they are written down, they are more likely to happen. These goals can be very enlightening for self-analysis.

Marge, a patient of mine, wrote a list of her goals about a year before she and her husband retired. They wrote their goals on a sheet of paper from a yellow legal pad and stuck the paper into the upper left hand slot of her big rolltop desk. When retirement came, she had pretty much forgotten about the list. She and her husband were busy building their dream home in a retirement community, on a beautiful hillside overlooking a lake.

At first they were very busy, and the adjustment to retirement living was not hard. But once the house was finished, and they had returned from some traveling they had planned to do, she began to feel alone and depressed. She couldn't understand why she would feel that way as it seemed that she had everything she had ever wanted.

Then, one night she was sitting alone in the den—her husband had gone to bed—and she happened to see the yellow piece of paper sticking out of the slot on the roll top desk, where it had been placed several years previously. She took it down and began to read the words she had written earlier about her goals of retirement. She realized that she had not met the goals she had planned at all! The goals she had planned had to do with what she wanted to be as a person, not with the material things that she wanted to possess.

No wonder she was not happy! She was off course! Her goals included such things as, "I want to be a loving, supportive wife. I want to be a good Christian. I want to be an example to my children and grandchildren."

"By reading these statements," she said, "I realized I was totally off base from what I really wanted. It was clear why I was depressed. From that moment on I read my list of goals every day and shared them with my husband. We moved back near our family and friends, and are now spending our money in the way we want to, rather than simply to have things. I am back on track with my life, and I am loving it!"

The written word is a stabilizing force in our lives. Many Vintage People have learned the power in this simple act. It is another characteristic that we can develop as we strive to become Vintage. According to Rollo May, "The more self-awareness a person has the more alive he is." Writing down personal goals and general philosophies of life is one way Vintage People remain self-aware and in harmony with the purpose of their lives.

One Vintage Person I know has accomplished an amazing string of good things in her life. The key to it all, she says, is to prepare our lives so that coincidence, good luck, and mystery can be welcomed and work for us. As she stated it, "If you want your ship to come in, then build an impressive dock for it!" Once the ship is in, then know how to enjoy what you have.

Self-esteem

It is not only our job to know ourselves, but also to correctly and realistically appraise ourselves. That can be hard to do. In medicine the old saying is correct: "He who treats himself has a fool for a patient!" It is much easier to evaluate another person or to diagnose another patient than to judge yourself without bias. Benjamin Franklin said, "There are three things extremely hard: steel, a diamond, and to know one's self!" God has given us a little ball of clay to live in, and it is difficult to get outside of it enough to be objective about ourselves.

Two dangers exist in the realm of self-esteem. The most common one is to undervalue ourselves. The other extreme is self righteousness or arrogance—overvaluing ourselves or thinking more highly of ourselves than we should. Both extremes will severely stifle us from becoming Vintage People. If we do the self-evaluation that I have suggested, and decide that we are truly better than most everyone else, we have not been realistic in our evaluation. If after self-evaluation we began to feel inferior and develop low self-esteem, we will never achieve Vintage Status.

Robert Schuller has a catchy saying that's worth thinking about: "You are not what you think you are, you are not what I think you are, you are what you think I think you are!"

That's pretty deep. Read it again! The best example I can think of to illustrate this point is an embarrassing story that happened to me a couple of years ago. At that time, I gave a talk to our local Lamaze classes about every six weeks. One night in particular I really seemed to be in the groove. The audience was laughing wholeheartedly at all my jokes and seemed to really be paying attention. My self-esteem soared as I perceived that I was doing a fantastic job! Afterwards I was really feeling good about myself. Then I discovered that my fly had been unzipped the entire lecture! "Why didn't you tell me?" I shrieked to the instructor.

"Oh," she replied, "I thought it was pretty funny, too!"

The high self-esteem that I was feeling came not from what the instructor thought of me, not from what the audience really thought of me; but from what I thought the audience thought of me. If I hadn't discovered the wayward zipper, I probably would still feel pretty good about that particular lecture. From that time forward, checking the zipper is the last thing I do before speaking to any group. I have learned from that mishap and have become more of a Vintage Person.

I've asked Vintage People how they learned to evaluate themselves in a practical, realistic way. After all, you can never please everyone nor conform to everyone's ideas.

Most relied only superficially upon other people's opinions. "I consider what my good friends and the people I respect think of me," says an eighty-eight-year-old salesman. "But I never listen to strangers because they don't know me!"

Another lady responded, "If you start to feel that you are better than someone else, you are wrong! If you start to feel inferior to someone else you are wrong! I've always used that as a guide, and it has served me very well."

Rather than depend upon others to judge their character, Vintage People rely more upon their own abilities. They know when they are right and often stick with it even if others mock them. They set their own standards to be judged by. I'm always inspired when I read of how famous people were often misjudged by the people around them. When Thomas Edison was seven years old, a school teacher gave him up as a hopeless case. In the boy's presence, the teacher told an inspector that Edison was "retarded" and that it was useless for him to attend school any longer. What would that do to one's self esteem?

A teacher is said to have written on a report about Abraham Lincoln: "When you consider that Abe has had only four months of school, he is very good with his studies, but he is a daydreamer and asks foolish questions."

Another authority wrote about Amelia Earhart, the pioneer aviatrice—"I am very concerned about Amelia. She is bright and full of curiosity, but her interest in bugs and other crawling things and her dare-devil projects are just not fitting for a young lady. Perhaps we could channel her curiosity into a safe hobby."

And my favorite of all time was written by a teacher about Albert Einstein. "Albert is a very poor student. He is mentally slow, unsociable, and is always daydreaming. He is spoiling it for the rest of the class. It would be in the best interests of all if he were removed from school at once."

Michael Jordan's high school coach cut him from the school basketball team. Dr. Seuss's first children's book was rejected by twenty-three publishers before the twenty-fourth sold six million copies. The Coca-Cola company sold only 400 Cokes their first year of business, and investors told them they had a product that would never "catch on!" And when Walt Disney submitted his first drawings for publication, the editor told him he had no artistic talent!

Each of these people realized early in life how to judge themselves. They trusted themselves and realized that even authority figures were not the determiners of their destinies. Rather, they themselves were. They set their own standards by which to be judged. They had that quality inherent in Vintage People to hold themselves accountable to a higher level. They realized that success may mean different things to different people. Only they can judge whether or not they are successful.

The importance of proper self-esteem was emphasized by one Vintage Patient I interviewed. To demonstrate what she meant, she enclosed the following verse from a poem called "The Person in the Glass," by an unknown author. I think it explains this characteristic better than any other example. Think of looking at yourself in a mirror:

"For it isn't your father or mother or mate,
Whose judgment upon you must pass;
The one whose verdict counts most in your life,
Is the one staring back from the glass."

Knowing others

In addition to understanding themselves fully, Vintage People have learned to know other people as well. Sociologists claim that eighty-five percent of the joy and satisfaction we get from life comes from interaction with other people.

Eighty-five percent! That means that only fifteen percent of our happiness comes from other sources: our garden, our yard, our dog, our money, and our possessions. That is why the Ebenezer Scrooges of this world end up so lonely and unhappy. They emphasize the wrong things in life and never become Vintage People.

Our ability to get along with others is of uttermost importance to our overall happiness. Vintage People learn the laws of human relationships somewhere along their sojourn in life. They do not isolate themselves. They do not count their worldly possessions greater than their relationships with others. They learn to value people and be genuinely interested in them.

In my line of work I often get the privilege—yes, I consider it a privilege—to be with patients and families at the time of death. So far, I've never heard a dying patient say, "I wish I had spent more time at the office! I wish I had a bigger house! I wish I had more money in my bank account!"

No! At that time of dimming life, material things seem much less important. I hear dying patients say things like, "I wish I could have spent more time with my children!" "I'm so glad we took that trip last spring!" "I am so fortunate to have so many people who love me!" "I wish I had worked less and loved more." "I'm so glad we spent the money to buy airline tickets for the whole family to be together last Christmas." When it comes right down to basic life, the majority of our pleasures of living involve relationships with other people.

But we are talking about self-esteem. How does this affect our relationships with other people? It is everything! Psychologists know that our own self-esteem has everything to do with how we get along with others. What we think of ourselves is of paramount importance in how we relate to others.

If we have high self-esteem—if we really like ourselves, we will get along with more people. People with low self-esteem function poorly with other people. They may be able to amass a fortune in earthly goods, but when they die they leave it all to their cat!

A corollary to this is the fact that people with the highest self-esteem will get along not only with the largest group of people, but they will get along well with the most diverse group of people as well. That is, it doesn't add much to our satisfaction with relationships if we only get along with those people that are like us. It is easy to like those who like us or have a lot in common with us. Only with a much more Vintage, or mature, attitude can we get along with people who are different from ourselves.

People of different professions, age groups—teenagers, children, and the elderly—races, and religions all have something to offer the Vintage Person. The measure of our healthy self-esteem, a healthy personality, is directly proportionate to the variety of diverse groups of people that we can befriend. The opposite is also true. Those who can get along with a limited number of people have a less healthy personality. Those who cannot get along with anyone have the least healthy personalities of all and usually live the life of a recluse, or spend their time in a mental institution or prison.

I have watched how Vintage People get along with others. They have learned some very important traits that make it easy. "Always smile," explained one Vintage Lady, "That makes the other person feel accepted." Other comments included: "Pay attention!" "Listen to the other person." "Give sincere compliments." "Be thankful and show appreciation." "Treat others the way you want to be treated."

Without knowing it, these Vintage People are using one of the mental laws that psychologists call the Law of Indirect Effort. That is, much of what we want in relationships comes to us in an indirect manner. For example, the best way to impress someone is to be impressed by them. If we want someone to like us, we must like them. To have someone respect us, we have to respect them. The best way to be trusted, is to trust. The best way to make a friend, as Emerson says, is to be a friend. God blesses us as we seek to bless others! The Law of Indirect Effort is one of the characteristics Vintage People have incorporated into their relationships in life.

How does this Law of Indirect Effort influence the self-esteem of Vintage People? It is simple! A classy ninety-year-old lady explained it to me like this: "Everyone thinks less of themselves than they ought to. I've found that when you build them up, you build yourself up, too!" Read that statement again! That is probably the most important concept humans can learn about building their own self-esteem.

This lady didn't read this fact in a self-help book or in a text of psychology, but she is describing another well-known scientific principle. The fact is that everybody has a self-esteem that is lower than it needs to be, from the greatest person on down. Who doesn't like to be built up? Husbands and wives especially can use this canon. As P.T. Forsyth explains it, "Love loves to be told what it knows already....It wants to be asked for what it longs to give."

Building someone up—if it is sincere and not just superficial flattery—is never wasted. That which is freely given, comes back. Shakespeare wrote it eloquently when he said, "The fragrance of the rose lingers on the hand that cast it!"

This is the rest of the story! Building someone else's self-esteem has tremendous benefits to the one doing the building. One of the greatest miracles of being human is that we *cannot* do anything to raise the self-esteem of another person, without raising our own self-esteem. Think about that! When we build others up, we paradoxically build ourselves up. What a wonderful way for this to work!

The ancients didn't know about the word "self-esteem," but they did understand this area of human relations. The Bible emphasizes this over and over: "Love your neighbor as yourself." "Do unto others as you would have them do unto you." "Go the second mile." "Turn the other cheek." The Bible is full of laws of human relationships involving self-esteem.

What would the world be like if it was the other way around? What if you could tear someone else down and build yourself up at the same time? Aren't we lucky that this cannot happen? Vintage People have learned that when they tear someone else down, they tear themselves down as well. This is a law of human psychology that works, just like the law of gravity works in the physical universe. As Martin Luther King said, "Everybody can be great because anybody can serve!"

What King meant by serving was doing things to make other people feel important. And the opposite is true—not doing things that make others feel unimportant. Without exception, when I brought this question before the Vintage People whom I interviewed, they summed it up by saying, "Follow the Golden Rule." That is exactly what Christ was telling His followers when He said, "And as you wish that men would do to you, do so to them."

Likewise, I think this principle is what Doctor Luke had in mind when he recorded Jesus' words in his Gospel: "Never criticize or condemn—or it will all come back on you. Go easy on others; then they will do the same for you. For if you give, you will get! Your gift will return to you in full and overflowing measure, pressed down, shaken together to make room for more, and running over. Whatever measure you use to give—large or small—will be used to measure what is given back to you." (Luke 6:37-38, *The Living Bible*)

FIVE

THE DISCIPLINED LIFE

*"Be bold in what you stand for and careful
what you fall for!"*

—Ruth Boorstin

One unexpected characteristic of Vintage People was revealed not by the responses they gave in their letters and interviews but by the very fact that they responded. I was amazed to get one hundred percent acknowledgment for the written requests I made. Those who were unable to write called or made a special visit to give me their thoughts personally.

When I first entertained the idea of sending out letters to Vintage People and asking for their insight about successful aging, I had two fears. I was apprehensive that I might offend them by implying that they were old, or that they might not want to take the time and effort to respond. After all, I was asking for considerable thought on their part. I'm not sure that I would like to be bothered with such an uninvited project. I was amazed at the results!

Within a few days of sending out the letters, my mailbox began to overflow! I found that neither of my worries was founded. First of all, they already knew they were old and readily accepted that fact. And to my amazement, they were happy to share their views and were flattered that someone had asked. Many actually thanked me for asking.

Irene, a retired nurse wrote, "Your letter arrived on a day when I needed a lift—the day before my eighty-first birthday. Eighty-one sounds so old, yet I am always happy to reach another birthday."

Oscar, who remains active in our community even as he enters his eighth decade of living, began his letter by expressing thanks, "I feel honored to receive your letter and hope I can help in some small way."

And Lillian, who at eighty-four continues to work part time in a local drugstore and spends the rest of her time going to her grandchildren's ball games, begins her reply— "I am so flattered that you included me in your study on aging. I only hope I can contribute in some small way." She sent me four very neatly typewritten pages of well-organized information that was extremely well thought out.

As I reflected on the overwhelming response to my letter, I began to realize that their willingness to respond was in itself one of the characteristics of Vintage People. No one had just thrown the letter aside and forgotten it. They had the self-discipline and courtesy to answer promptly and politely. They were willing to share with others of their experience and knowledge, and they were thankful to have the opportunity to do so.

What better set of circumstances could we as a younger generation take advantage of than this great wealth of knowledge and experience in a group of Vintage People who are delighted to share it!

We often go to classes, counselors and attend seminars, spending large amounts of money, for the kind of practical information that Vintage People offer for free. We are missing a tremendous opportunity when we fail to take advantage of this situation. And likewise, we can learn from the disciplines that they have built into their lives.

Integrity

A psychologist I heard speak some time ago made a simple statement that caught my attention. I had never thought about it before, but it is absolutely true. He said, "Practically 100 percent of the patients who I counsel come to me because of distressed relationships. And their problems usually exist because one or more of the people involved have treated someone badly."

Relationships! I must admit that I have never referred anyone to a psychologist because of a problem with his car, because the sewer backed up at home, or because there was water in a person's basement. Those things may seem important at the time and cause some stress, but they are disabling only when they also disrupt human relationships. Relationships make up the most important part of life. In addition, relationships can become so strained that we are unable to deal with the other aspects of life, and the joy of living is gone.

When relationships go wrong the impact can devastate our whole being. Troubles in this area can affect performance at work, sleeping and eating habits, physical health, and finally a person's happiness and ability to function. We can't perform well when the significant relationships in our lives are faulty. We must get along well with people to be happy. That means treating others well.

In my research I found Vintage People repeating one concept of relationships. It may sound simple, but they have arrived at this idea first hand though trial and error. A great number of Vintage People believe in, and try to live by, the "Golden Rule." That is: "Do unto others as you would have them do unto you." If you think about it, that pretty much covers human relationships. It's that simple! Albert Einstein said that the statement, "Love thy neighbor as thyself," is "…like a natural law almost like a physical part of the universe."

I believe that successful "loving" of yourself and your neighbor goes even deeper. Vintage People tell me it also involves a quality that I can only call "integrity." Integrity means doing the "right thing." It means doing the right thing even when it is hard. It means doing the right thing even when no one is looking, and no one will ever find out.

There is a certain stop light in the town where I practice that I have to pass on the way to the hospital. In our small town there is seldom much traffic after midnight. While on my way to the hospital at three o'clock in the morning, I have often contemplated not stopping for that red light. I can easily see that there is no traffic in either direction. I can also easily observe that no police cars are in sight! Yet I usually stop and sit there, waiting for the green light and feeling kind of foolish since I am the only car for blocks around. While lightheartedly discussing this one day, I was delighted and relieved to find out that my partners do the same thing! We concluded that we are all compulsive, but we have integrity!

I am thrilled that medical science is beginning to recognize the value of integrity in relationships as well as in our mental and physical health. When I was in medical school, these ideas would have been rapidly dismissed as being "in the realm of religion." But as the study of science is bringing us back to the importance of religion, integrity is currently recognized by clinicians to be important. Some psychologists now even have a mode of treatment called "Integrity Therapy." Simply stated, this theory suggests that most emotional and mental illnesses come from our disobedience to what Carl Jung calls the "Universal Subconscious." Steve Covey calls it the "Universal Moral Sense of all Mankind."

Whether you look at it from a religious perspective or from a scientific viewpoint, and no matter what you call it, human beings seem to possess an inherent knowledge of "right and wrong." This force is strong in our lives. Vintage People have learned that they cannot be happy as long as they are at odds with this basic moral conscious. They have learned that they cannot live a lie. They must "come clean." Violation of our conscience will lead to anxiety, stress, unhappiness, and eventually to mental and physical health problems.

Josh Billings says, "One of the greatest victories you can gain over someone is to beat him at politeness." This "game" really works! We teach our receptionists to be polite from their first day. The best way to handle an irate patient is to smile and be sickeningly polite. It not only disarms the angry person, but it also helps the receptionist keep her cool. King Solomon wrote, "If your enemy is hungry, give him bread to eat; and if he is thirsty, give him water to drink; for you will heap coals of fire on his head, and the Lord will reward you."

Of course, this is easier said than done! One of the great privileges I enjoy as a family physician is watching family dynamics. Sometimes it is good and rewarding; sometimes it is disastrous. But it is always insightful! Some people have very elaborate rationalization systems. And they may be able to fool everyone else, but they can never fool themselves. I've seen a lot of Non-vintage People try to do just that. I've seen teenagers turn their backs on family values and get involved in all kinds of mischief. I've even seen some run away from home and marry someone who is dependent upon alcohol, or into drugs, or is abusive to them. I've watched as those marriages become strained and often collapse under the stress and anxiety of the situation. Why? Because the victim was not in harmony with his or her conscience. Eventually, they could not change and live in violation of their own conscience, and the situation becomes intolerable. In *The Turquoise Lament,* John D. MacDonald describes integrity this way: "Integrity is not a conditional word. It doesn't blow in the wind or change with the weather. It is your inner image of yourself, and if you look in there and see a man who won't cheat, then you know he never will."

I've treated the middle-aged male or female who is having an affair and living a lie. In spite of all the rationalization that takes place consisting of all the resources that success may have brought him or her, after awhile the situation becomes unbearable. Often the whole circumstance explodes. Sometimes, however, I have seen my patients suddenly decide to "come clean." I have marveled at the therapeutic value of that. Once they reach that stage, I know they are cured. They will usually describe a tremendous "peace," even though they may have more work to do in their lives than ever.

Any physician will tell you that a large number of patients who come to the office do not have any real physical disease. Most medical doctors are pretty good at spotting these patients. I recently saw a middle-aged lady with a number of complaints, none of which fit into the pattern of any disease that I knew. I don't pretend to know all the rare conditions that afflict people, but I do have a sense of which patients have something physical. And this lady was very high on the "crock" scale.

Falling into the usual scientific doctor mode, I ordered the standard battery of tests. Of course, they were all normal. One important clue that helps confirm my suspicions that I'm dealing with psychological rather than physical problems occurs when the patient returns to review his laboratory work with me. I purposely do not start the visit by showing the test results. I usually inquire how they've been doing since the last office visit. If they fail to ask about their test results, I begin to suspect the problem is not physical. After all, if you are really worried about a physical ailment, you will be anxious to find out what the doctor has discovered.

This lady followed the pattern that I expected. On the second visit she did not ask about her test results. I theorize that this is because these patients sub-consciously know that the results will be normal. On her return visit, rather than acknowledging the lab work that had been done, she immediately went into an extensive list of new symptoms she had prepared for me.

At that point it was obvious to me that if I was going to help this patient at all, I was going to have to stop re-enforcing her health concerns with further laboratory tests and explore what was really going on in her life. When she was about twenty minutes into her ten-minute office call, and about a third of the way through her list, I interrupted her. "Mary," I said. "All these symptoms are overwhelming my mind. You must really feel horrible trying to live with all this. I certainly need to know how you are handling this in your life. For example, how are things between you and your husband?"

She immediately broke into tears! "We have been like stranger for years. I was so lonely until I met Sam. He was the first man to listen to me in years."

Well, one thing had led to another, and she had been having an affair for about nine months. "At first I really liked the excitement, and I was just sure I could hide it from my husband, and have the best of both worlds. And it is working. No one knows, and my husband doesn't suspect a thing. So it seems I should be happy! But I am so miserable I want to die!" Finally she was able to pull herself together a little, and she asked, "Do you think that is what is affecting my health?"

The answer was obvious. I explained to her the idea of integrity therapy. Even though she had done an excellent job of rationalizing and had fooled everyone else, she could not fool her own sense of right and wrong. The process was literally making her sick! A very long list of sick!

An approach like this doesn't always work, but this person seemed to understand what I was telling her. I was able to get her into counseling with a friend of mine who also uses a direct approach. The story has a happy ending. I saw her about a month later for an insurance physical. I was surprised at how much calmer and at peace she seemed. I didn't bring up our former conversation, but she did.

"Doctor," she began, "I want to let you know I have solved that list of problems I had!"

"Yes," I replied. "You seem to be feeling very well."

"I really am," she continued. "I knew I had to get Sam out of my life, and I did it. My husband still doesn't know any of this, but he has agreed that our marriage isn't what it used to be, and he has agreed to work on it with me. I am so happy—and I really feel good physically, too." This lady was demonstrating what Nathaniel Hawthorne was talking about when he wrote, "No man, for any considerable time, can wear one face to himself and another to the multitude without finally getting bewildered as to which may be the true!"

Vintage People have learned that by practicing integrity they can be in accord with the universal moral sense. They live with integrity. They live with discipline. But let me make something very clear. I'm not saying that a Vintage Person has to fit a certain mold. They do not need to be "stuffy" in their disciplined life. Living the disciplined life is not stifling. It is really just the opposite! Once they have discovered how to do the "right thing," and to live with integrity, tremendous freedoms are theirs to enjoy. Good things tend to flow towards them. It is almost as though they are in tune with the universe and joys abound. Of course, even Vintage People occasionally miss the mark a little. When that happens, the "moral laws of the universe" will call them back to the disciplined life. Vintage People become skilled at listening to these laws. They become sensitive to feeling what the world is feeding them.

Again, let me stress that my investigations with Vintage People have made it clear that I cannot sell any specific life-style here. I'm not saying that Vintage People have to look like this or that! Everyone has a true self that must be developed. The world would not want it any other way. The point is that Vintage People recognize that they must live the truth. This involves living with integrity. They cannot fool themselves, and when they try, they don't feel as sound mentally or physically. One Vintage Man stated it like this: "I have learned to listen to the still, small voice of my conscience, and not to talk back to it!"

Reasons

Ask a teenager what he or she did at school today. The answer you will invariably get is, "Nothing!" What are you going to do tomorrow? "I don't know!" How long have you been sick? "I don't know!" The answer you generally get for almost everything is, "I don't know!" Early in my medical practice I was somewhat offended when adolescents would answer my medical questions that way while I was trying to get their medical history. I feared they either didn't like me, or they didn't trust me with their medical information. But then I discovered, they are being truthful!

They really don't know! There are so many things that either they haven't ever thought about or just haven't made up their minds about.

Contrast this with Vintage People. Ask Vintage People why they believe a certain way, or why they do certain things, and they can give you the reason. They seldom say, "I don't know!" Vintage People have formed an opinion on almost everything in life, from health matters to UFOs to why they always start shaving on the same side of their face each morning. They have an explanation for everything! Superficially, this seems to make sense. As we mature we encounter more situations, have had a chance to think about more things, and learn more of what does and does not work in life.

Ronald Reagan was beyond the customary retirement age when he ran for re-election as US President in 1984. During the televised debate between Reagan and Walter Mondale, a reporter asked Reagan if he was too old for another term. "I'm not going to inject the issue of age into this campaign," he said. "I am not going to exploit for political gain my opponent's youth and inexperience!"

Vintage People have valuable experience, but not all Vintage People draw the same conclusions from the same evidence. I noticed this first in regard to health matters such as diet. My older patients would often say "I don't eat that." When asked why, they always had a reason. "It upsets my stomach!" "I read that it's not good for you!" "My great Aunt ate that and had to have bowel surgery the next day!" One gentleman told me, "A hog won't eat a cucumber, and I make it a rule never to eat something a pig won't eat!" Whether it was a reason I agreed with or not, they still had a reason—something that they had learned by trial and error, by experience!

Other health habits had the same basis in experience. If a patient explained that he or she always did certain exercises before going to bed, they knew why. Perhaps it helped them sleep better. If they drank wine with a meal, it helped their digestion. Warm milk before bedtime helped them rest. Prune juice every morning helped with their bowels and thus their health. Benjamin Franklin found that if he undressed in a cold room and waited until he was shivering and could not stand the cold any longer, he could then jump into bed, pull the covers up and quickly go to sleep as the warmth returned to his body.

My point here is not the specific little quirks that people have developed, but that they have developed them because of logically perceived reasons. I'm not going to judge whether or not their reasons are correct scientifically or medically, and not all reasons work for all people, but if they are believed then they work for that particular person. Ask Vintage People their opinion on politics or the controversial social issues of the day. If they give you an opinion, they will know why they believe as they do. If they haven't thought it through thoroughly, they are not afraid to tell you, "I haven't decided yet."

This ability to make decisions and form opinions based upon reason seems to be a very important factor in maturity and in believing in yourself. As a young medical student I felt unsure because I didn't understand all the reasons why my attending physicians were doing certain things. Gradually I reached the point where I knew the reason for each test, each X-ray, and each statement made to a patient. I gained confidence which made me a more competent physician. Vintage People have gained that same confidence about life. They understand the reasons for things. This characteristic can come only through experience, through learning, and then through the discipline to follow what they have learned.

Self-discipline

In response to my questions and letters, almost all of the Vintage People listed diet and exercise as two characteristics that helped them achieve their status. I suspect one reason for the popularity of that answer was the fact that I am a physician. They probably felt I wanted to hear that! And, of course I do feel that both are important.

It wasn't until I asked a few more questions that I began to have some doubts—especially about diet. Exercise, it seems, was pursued to about the same degree for everyone. Exercise mostly involved walking followed by working outside, gardening, climbing stairs, or housework. We will talk specifically about exercise later. Diet puzzled me. One very sharp eighty-eight-year-old suggested drinking three glasses of milk each day. Another active lady who continues to sing at numerous functions states that she has never consumed milk or milk products. Several people mentioned eating fruits and vegetables, but when really quizzed about it, admitted that they eat only one or two servings per day—which is below the US Government's recommended guidelines. Another gentleman who seems to have an endless supply of energy states he "...avoids greasy foods, but I do like sweets. I never skip desserts!" Others avoid sugar at all costs.

Another active lady sent me literature on the importance of eating garlic every day! One attributed her longevity to consuming a teaspoon of vinegar every morning and every evening! Some felt that fiber was vital to their diet; others skipped all fiber. Some were heavy coffee drinkers; others never drank it. Some drank several bottles of Pepsi or Coke every day; others drank only water. Some of the Vintage People were teetotalers; others had one or two drinks with their meals. None drank excessively. Only a couple were smokers, but there were a large number who had been smokers and had quit.

When I got to these statistics, my scientific brain thought, "How am I going to make any significant conclusions about the importance of diet?" There was no pattern! The dietary habits of Vintage People were as diverse as their personalities.

However, I knew that there is often a pattern even in chaos. I began to see a common thread. Perhaps it wasn't the diet itself that was responsible for their long quality of life, but the fact that they were disciplined enough to follow a diet consistently. The fact that a number of these people were ex-smokers showed that they have a great amount of will power—that they have discipline. Maybe this is the characteristic that I was looking for rather than the magic component of their diet. Vintage People seem to have the discipline to follow a specific diet well. After all, it takes a fair amount of discipline to swallow a teaspoon of vinegar every night and morning!

They have the discipline to exercise in whatever fashion it may be. They have the discipline to stop smoking when the evidence on the dangers of tobacco became known. This is a disciplined group of folks! They are strict on themselves. This characteristic carries over into other aspects of their lives. Listen to the resourcefulness that one Vintage Lady has used to discipline herself to exercise. "Exercise has always been a must for me even though I often have to resort to tricking myself into it—such as intentionally leaving things upstairs necessitating extra trips up and down. I like to park my car a distance from my destination and walk. I try to use the stairs rather than the elevator. I really believe the old saying, 'If you don't use it—you lose it!'" Now that requires self discipline!

Vintage People show discipline in many other ways. They are on time. They pay their bills. They follow schedules—Vintage People are the only ones who show up for their appointments when the Kansas snowstorms come; the younger people all cancel! Vintage People keep promises. They are disciplined in their finances, often living on a fixed income. They are disciplined in their spiritual and prayer life. They don't give into "peer" pressure. They don't do things that are against their integrity or beliefs. They work at controlling their tempers. They work at forgiving and being flexible. And they accept the consequences when self-discipline fails them.

I recently visited the winter homes of Thomas Edison and Henry Ford in Fort Meyers, Florida. Although these two gentlemen were good friends, they had very different attitudes about life-styles. Thomas Edison felt the body was only good to carry the brain around. He never exercised, ate what he wanted, and smoked cigars. Henry Ford was a teetotaler, watched his diet closely, and believed in the benefits of exercise—he was an avid square dancer and walker. Thomas Edison died at age 83 and Henry Ford at the age of 84! So we are left to draw our own conclusions about life style.

But the one thing that both of these great Americans had in common was discipline. They were both extremely disciplined people. It appears that the characteristic of discipline is what we are looking for here. The specifics of that discipline may vary, but Vintage People all seem to possess a large amount of self-control. Listen to a few more disciplines from Vintage People.

From an eighty-plus-year-old who continues to teach a college class for older adults, "I have learned to discipline myself and not let TV absorb my time. I turn the TV way down and the book reading way up!"

Another Vintage Lady responds, "It is a self-discipline of mine to get dressed, make-up on and my hair combed, and be ready for the day as soon as possible after I arise each morning. I find that to be a true morale booster."

And finally, listen to the discipline, and the beauty, in this statement from a seventy-seven-year-old interim minister. "It has been my habit each day upon awakening to ask God to guide me through the day and show me how I can use my life to share with others, whom He has created in such a special way. God did not create me to hibernate nor to live in isolation. I have disciplined myself to affirm life."

The discipline of forgiveness

Vintage People have learned it is not in their best interest to carry a grudge. Stated another way, Vintage People seem to be very forgiving. They have learned a great principle of life. Carrying a grudge or failing to forgive is a major roadblock to happiness and success. Jesus taught this fact of human interaction two thousand years ago. Mahatma Gandhi taught, "The weak can never forgive. Forgiveness is the attitude of the strong." Today's psychologists are just now re-discovering the power of forgiveness. We forgive another, not for their sake, but for our own sake. It may seem ironic, but forgiving someone makes the forgiver feel good, whether or not it helps the one who is forgiven.

I treated a patient a number of years ago for chronic ulcers and high blood pressure. As a young and eager physician I remember trying all the scientific and pharmaceuticals at my disposal. Nothing seemed to work. Dan seemed to be getting worse in spite of my best efforts. I

am a medical doctor, not a psychiatrist. I don't necessarily
believe that every illness has some sort of psychological
basis, but in desperation I decided to probe into his personal life a little further.

What I found was astonishing. After I had gained his
confidence, he shared with me something that was literally
eating him alive. It seems he had worked diligently on a
project for his company for several years sacrificing everything. But just when he was ready to present the project
which he was sure would gain him a large promotion and
raise, one of his most trusted co-workers stole his project
and submitted it as his own. He stole his ideas and took
credit for them. Even worse was the fact that this co-
worker was given a big raise and was promoted to be my
patient's boss. Every day now he had to go to work and follow orders from someone who had betrayed him.

As this story finally poured forth, I could visualize my
patient's blood pressure climbing, and the stomach acid
churning out. I inquired about changing jobs, which he
could not do. Finally I said, "Dan, you are just going to
have to forgive him and go on with your life!"

He said I didn't understand and that he would never be
happy until he had his revenge. Then he stormed out of the
office, and I was sure I had said the wrong thing. I didn't
see him again for several years and figured he had changed
to another doctor who was less prone to give him a Sunday
school lesson for his physical illness.

One day he called and wanted me to have lunch with
him. I learned he had just bought the company where he
worked. As the new owner, he wanted me to be their medical director. While visiting over lunch I had an opportunity
to find out what really had happened—the rest of the story.

He had indeed changed doctors and had gotten much
worse. He had been hospitalized in another city with bleed-

ing ulcers. He told me, "While lying in that hospital bed, not knowing whether or not I was going to have to have surgery, or maybe even bleed to death, your words came back to me. For the first time I realized that my obsession with resentment and revenge was literally eating me alive! I decided that no matter what, I had to forgive that SOB for my own good. He had stolen my project, and now he was going to steal my health, my happiness, and maybe even my life as well!"

"It was hard," he continued. "But almost immediately after making that decision, I began to feel better, both physically and mentally. I actually began to be courteous and helpful to my boss. It was so amazing! Suddenly I recognized an opportunity that had been staring me in the face for years. I just hadn't been able to see it because of my obsession on getting even and being hurt so badly.

"By seeing this opportunity I was able to raise the money to actually buy the company. The one that had hurt me so much got his money and was on his way. And I didn't even feel resentful about it. Even though I am working harder than ever now, I feel great. I eat anything I want to, and my blood pressure is back to normal without medications."

Vintage People seem to have learned this lesson well. They are very forgiving—whether they recognize it or not—for their own well-being. They have the ability to put all sorts of bad things behind them, forgive, and go on with their lives. My patient, Dan, is on his way to someday becoming a Vintage Person. Mark Twain put it elegantly when he wrote, "Forgiveness is the fragrance the violet sheds on the heel that has crushed it."

It is all a part of the disciplined life!

SIX

FLEXIBILITY

"The really happy person is the one who can enjoy
the scenery
when he has to take a detour."

—Unknown

Life is a great teacher," states a ninety-three-year-old
great-grandmother, "and one of the lessons it has taught me
is to be flexible. I try to look at all sides of something before
making up my mind. The more I've lived, the more I've
learned to never judge someone else!"

Vintage People are not inflexible. They seem to have
reached a time in their lives where they are more flexible,
more tolerant of others, and very non-judgmental. I'm not
sure where this originates, but it seems to be the result of
accepting people as they are. Vintage People have learned
to accept and treasure the differences in people. They
somehow expect people to be human and to make mistakes. When others do make mistakes, it doesn't bother
them much.

I first discovered this characteristic of Vintage People
when working with adolescents, some of the most challenging patients a physician will ever treat. I remember
some of them vividly. One patient I saw first when she was
fifteen years old. I had the additional advantage as a family physician to know her parents as well. They seemed to
be a stable, well-adjusted family. But their daughter was

83

going through a very turbulent time in her life, with disorders such as bulimia, promiscuous behavior, and drug and alcohol experimentation. It was somewhat of a surprise to me that this fifteen-year-old trusted me enough to tell me her problems. I was careful not to do anything to betray her trust and never related any of this to her parents, as she requested me not to.

In working with her problems, I felt she needed someone to talk to and suggested she talk with her parents, or at least her mother, a school counselor, or some other trusted adult. She felt she could not do this. Then I found, much to my surprise, that she had a grandmother with whom she had been talking. It turned out that her grandmother was the one who had convinced her to confide in me.

"Why did you choose your grandmother to trust?" I asked her.

"Because my grandmother is so cool!" she replied.

As I got further into treating this young lady and counseling her, I, too, began to see how her grandmother was "so cool." First of all, my adolescent patient completely trusted her grandmother. She was confident that she could pour out her biggest hurts without the fear of reprisal or betrayal. That was essential, but grandmother's "coolness" went even deeper than that. Her grandmother took the time to listen and tried to understand. She was flexible. She did not approve of the behavior in which the girl was engaging, but she tried to understand and to look at all aspects of the situation.

But the biggest part of the "coolness," I believe, was the fact that her grandmother was not judgmental. She accepted her granddaughter as she was. She saw her as a fellow human, and as such she knew she would make mistakes. Her grandmother saw life as a teacher. She knew that her granddaughter was learning from her experiences—and sometimes an education can be expensive. She was showing unconditional love. She did not take the shortsighted view centering on the things my patient was doing wrong. She was seeing her as a whole person, with a long and good life ahead of her.

When I finally got a chance to talk to the grandmother about the help she was providing, all of the above characteristics were reconfirmed. "She is a good girl from a good family," she told me. "I know she will eventually get her direction straight and do okay. Right now I am just trying to support her and nudge her in the right direction. It won't all be done at once, but we will get there."

A Vintage Grandfather, a retired pilot, described it this way: "As a pilot I learned the importance of plotting a course to follow if you ever expected to get to your destination. But I have also learned to be flexible. Flying consists of a series of small corrections. At any time I try to be near my plotted course, but probably ninety percent of the time I am not exactly on course. But I remain flexible and keep making corrections."

"Life is a lot like flying," he continued. "I see that in my own life as well as others. I've always tried to keep my children and grandchildren near the proper course. As long as they are close, the corrections are easy to make. If they get off course further, they have larger adjustments to make in order to end up where they want to be. But in life, as in flying, there is no such thing as, 'you can't get there from here!' You may have to do some maneuvering, or even retrace your course—but if you know were you are going, you can always get there."

Vintage People do seem to live beyond themselves. They often are teachers who seem close to the truth. Maybe this comes only with maturity, but Vintage People seem to be a little more in touch with their feelings. They are more apt to think with their hearts than totally with their brains. I guess this makes sense, for if God put us here for any purpose, then there must be a point later in life where this begins to happen. Wordsworth says that children enter this world "trailing clouds of glory." Perhaps Vintage People also begin to approach spiritual truths as they near the end of this earthly journey and approach eternity from the other end.

Interruptions

Vintage People seem to know how to handle interruptions. Perhaps I should say they have learned the *value* of interruptions. They have a set routine in life but don't mind interruptions. A retired minister referred to interruptions as "blessed disturbances." One ninety-year-old lady told me, "Interruptions are the most memorable part of my life."

I wasn't sure what she meant until she explained. "I don't mean annoying interruptions—like phone salesmen. I mean quality interruptions such as when a friend drops by, when my grandchildren visit, or when someone in church taps me on the shoulder and tells me they are glad I'm there. Labor and childbirth was always a joyful interruption for me. And the times my children interrupted me to soothe their tears and to share their unexpected joys are the unplanned times that I remember most." (She raised eleven children, so you can imagine the interruptions she must have had!)

Thinking about this, I have concluded that we need to realize the greatness that often comes with interruptions. I used to get frustrated at the interruptions in my medical practice. It seemed the best planning went for naught. It never failed that on the busiest day in the office, I would be called to the delivery room or the emergency room.

But after talking to this wise Vintage Lady, I began to realize that as I looked back over the day, the week, and the year, it was precisely those pesky interruptions that I remembered. What could be more exciting than delivering a new life into this world and sharing that great joy with the new parents? And what about the man I had to see in the emergency room with the ruptured abdominal aneurysm? I still remember the flurry of activity as we got him stabilized and the Lifewatch helicopter flew him to the waiting surgical suite in our referral hospital. I remember the sense of pride when he had successful surgery there and returned to our town grateful to all of us.

I remember these events. But I don't remember the patients with routine appointments for blood pressure checks or "50,000 mile checkups" that I left behind. My office patients hate it, but I almost look forward to interruptions! Interruptions are often the best memories of life.

When you think about it, almost any change comes as an interruption to someone. Most events that have changed world history were interruptions from the routine. Scientists tell us that dinosaurs methodically ruled the earth for six hundred million years. Then one day an asteroid smashed into our planet, changing the climate so drastically that they could no longer survive. What an interruption!

World War II was an interruption in the lives of millions of people, but look how it changed human history. My mother was interrupted by labor pains when I was born— but I am grateful that it happened!

If we look at the lives of great people, the interruptions in their lives are often the best remembered. Some of the greatest miracles Jesus performed involved interruptions. He was traveling in a hurry when a centurion interrupted him to heal his servant. We remember the miracle of the healing, but we don't remember where Jesus was going or what he did once He got there. The feeding of the five thousand was an unplanned interruption. Jesus was seeking solitude after learning of the death of John the Baptist. The crowds followed Him to a lonely place—and didn't even bring any food! Even His arrest was an interruption of the

Passover festivities. That interruption changed civilization more than any other event in history.

Look how Moses' life was interrupted. And Noah's! The point is that the interruption is more important, more memorable, and more rewarding than day-to-day activities we are often so intent doing. Interruptions force us to "live in the moment." When interruptions come our way, we are compelled to trust that things will somehow work out. We cannot dwell on or worry about interruptions, but must simply make the best of them. Vintage People realize that interruptions are often opportunities. They are frequently the most challenging times of life. Some interruptions result in good memories, and some in bad ones—but they are memories. Many of the important things that happen to us come out of the blue as interruptions.

Age discrimination

Unfortunately, not all spheres requiring flexibility in the lives of Vintage People are positive. I found one area that drew negative comments from almost everyone I interviewed. This was the subject of age discrimination. Vintage People do not complain much about their health, nor about taxes, Social Security, or Medicare. There are things about each of these areas that they don't particularly like, but when I mentioned age discrimination, they all got, as one Vintage Grandmother put it, "fired up!"

How does American society respond to the wealth of information contained in the minds of our Vintage People? Unfortunately, we ignore it. We sometimes act like the "mindless stooge" described by C.S. Lewis who threw out all the vintage wine because it was old! What a waste of a valuable commodity!

Dr. Robert Butler, former head of the National Institute of Aging, states in his Pulitzer Prize winning book (*Aging and Mental Health: Positive Psychological and Biomedical Approaches*, 1998), "Old age is frequently a tragedy; even when the early years have been fulfilling and people seemingly have everything going for them. Herein lies what I consider to be the genuine tragedy of old age in America. We have shaped a society which is extremely harsh to live in when one is old."

One of my Medicare patients brought the whole arena of age discrimination to my attention. I guess I had never thought much about it—which indicates how big a problem it may be! Society expects older people to accept being discriminated against and to lose a lot of their freedoms of choice as they age.

For example, many people are forced into retirement. The assumption seems to be that as we age to about sixty-five years, we can no longer do the job we once did. I have spent considerable effort trying to discover exactly how the age of sixty-five became the benchmark of "old age." The historical facts will surprise you.

When Bismark was chancellor of Germany in the 1870s he noticed that all of his powerful and influential political enemies were men over the age of sixty-five. These were the Vintage People of the time who had gained enough wisdom and resources to challenge his leadership. Therefore, he convinced the German legislature to make age sixty-five the mandatory age for retirement and "old age." Ironically, the age of sixty-five had nothing to do with a person's drop in productivity or decline in their mental abilities. Just the opposite! It had to do with their power, wisdom, experience and organization. It had to do with all the positive things about aging that we have been describing in this book. This seems to be the model that the United States Social Security System adopted when it was established in 1935. The number "sixty-five" was chosen for all the wrong reasons!

Hence the stereotyping of old age began. Once someone reached this select age, they were old—according to the government and the nation's work force. Retirement was expected. Society felt that older people were not capable of deciding for themselves when retirement was appropriate—they needed a number. Therefore, mandatory retirement, based solely upon age, was born.

I have a Vintage Person in my practice who is an airline pilot with years of experience. He has never had any type of reportable accident and remains in excellent physical shape medically. However, upon reaching the age of sixty (the so-called age-sixty rule), he was required to step out of the cockpit for good. The day before his birthday he was competent to captain a 747 full of passengers into and out of Dallas/Fort Worth International Airport, but the day after his birthday he wasn't even allowed to taxi a plane on the ramp. This is unfortunately typical of many occupations and corporations. Only one thing is relevant—age: a number.

Discrimination is based on emotion or prejudice rather than scientific fact. If an airline pilot who turns sixty or even sixty-five years of age is a more dangerous pilot all of a sudden, then the practice of retiring pilots at that age is a good one. If it is based purely on generalization, a feeling, or someone's guess or perception, then it is blatant discrimination.

Do we have any scientific data showing that after sixty-five employees become a liability or a danger to themselves and others? Being an Airman Medical Examiner, I know the FAA, as well as the airline industry, has struggled with this question for years. Certainly a pilot's reflexes and physical strength may decrease with age. But these changes vary from person to person. No one would feel comfortable watching an elderly senile gentleman with thick glasses, hearing aids, and a walker, trying to find his way to the cockpit to pilot your plane across the country. But neither would I be comfortable with a twenty-five-year-old pilot if he had the same physical disabilities. The question is whether or not AGE itself is the major factor involved. If age is not the single reason that you would not want to fly with this person, then using age as an excuse to keep him out of the pilot's seat is discriminatory just as much as if we used skin color, sex or body habitus as an excuse to prevent someone from doing a certain task. Any time people are pre-judged because of some factor over which they have no control, whether it be age, race, sex, or religious origin, then their true worth is being overlooked, and we are wasting some of this country's resources.

Numerous "soft" discriminatory practices against age thrive in most social institutions, government, and even in medical care. In most government jobs, there is still a forced retirement age. True, governments and social organizations have developed "Senior Citizens Centers" over the country, but these are designed to entertain, or "care for" older people—not to draw strength from them! I have a vibrant ninety-six year-old-patient who refuses to go there. "There's just too many old people there," she tells me. And I think she is right! These institutions are not designed for creativity and the giving of positive benefits back to society. Even Medicare is discriminatory. Preventive medicine is not encouraged. The attitude seems to be that it is for "old people" anyway, so let's just spend as little as possible on medical care to get by until nature takes its course and they die.

This is the only negative section in this book. I thought seriously about leaving it out for that reason. I decided this is a topic Vintage People want the public to know about, and that the book would not be complete without mentioning it. When I began asking my Vintage Patients about age discrimination, I got a more emotional response than on any other subject! One patient commented, "Oh, Doc, you had better give me an extra blood pressure pill before I start!"

Everyone I asked was able to give me story after story of what they felt was age discrimination. Many mentioned that fact that they felt avoided by various merchants and salesclerks, particularly the younger ones. One feisty eighty-year-old told me she had heard a manager tell his salesgirl, "Go wait on those other people first. That old lady will take a long time to make up her mind, and she probably isn't going to buy very much anyway!" Needless to say, she didn't buy very much in that store! Ironically, that eighty-year-old Vintage Lady could have bought the entire store if she had wanted to!

Another Vintage Couple that I see regularly for their medical care come from another city about thirty miles away. That city is much bigger than where I practice and has many more doctors. I've always been curious as to why they choose to travel to my office. One day I asked if they had thought about what they would do if they had a medical emergency and needed care right away. They explained to me why they preferred my office.

"The doctors at home don't like old people," the wife clarified to me. "Our town has one major employer—an oil refinery. The people who work there have great insurance. The doctors don't want to see anyone who doesn't work there. Medicare does not pay enough."

"It probably just seems that way," I said, trying to stick up a little for the medical profession.

Her husband interrupted, "Let me tell you about the last time I tried to make an appointment there. I called the office and said I wanted to make an appointment. The office girl seemed friendly and interested. She took my name and the nature of my problem. Then she wanted to know which insurance I had. When I replied I was on Medicare, her tone suddenly changed. 'Doctor only takes a few new Medicare patients each week,' she told me. 'It will be about four to six weeks before we can squeeze you in. You may want to call another doctor's office!' I got a similar response at every office I called."

Sounds like discrimination, doesn't it? If this occurred because of race, skin color, or sex, it would be immoral, not to mention illegal. But in talking to Vintage People, discrimination is extremely common. It is another one of the things that Vintage People have accepted and learned to be flexible with. While Vintage People tolerate it, our country is failing to realize the full value of one of our most priceless assets.

Adaptation

Vintage People have found that they must be flexible, but they have also found that they can be *too* flexible. Just as there are dangers in being inflexible, there are also dangers in adapting too much. One Vintage Person stated it like this: "The old ways are not always the best! But, then, some of the new ways are not best either. At my age I've learned to not be wishy-washy. I don't overreact, but I also won't lower my standards!"

I remember a somewhat cruel experiment we did in one of my college classes that illustrates the danger of being too flexible, or too adaptive. While studying the life-style of frogs, our professor impressed upon us how adaptive these little green creatures were. They have survived over millions of years, even as the earth has changed. They have adapted to living in the water or on land. They can live in hot weather or cold weather. Even dry or wet climates don't bother them much. Biologically speaking, their survival has been attributed to this remarkable ability to adapt—to be flexible.

However, the experiment that the professor performed in class showed us the dangers of being over-adaptive. He placed several live frogs in a shallow pan of water at room temperature. The pan had no lid, so the frogs could jump out at any time if they wished. Then a Bunsen burner was started under the pan to slowly warm the water. True to their nature, the frogs adapted to the warming water and didn't even seem to notice that it was getting dangerously hot.

Fortunately, the professor stopped the experiment when the water was uncomfortably hot to human touch. But, the frogs just sat there content to adapt to their environment. The professor went on to explain that he could have kept heating the water and the frogs would have died. I have no reason to doubt his word. They were so flexible in adapting to their surroundings that they didn't notice what was gradually happening to them. Things were changing so much as to become dangerous to their very survival, but they paid no attention.

Vintage People have learned to not be that flexible. They have an ability to change and adapt when change is needed, but they always keep an eye on the "big picture" of what is going on around them. They select the areas where they are going to be flexible and the areas where they are going to stand firm. Just like the frogs, "taking a little heat" can be just fine, but Vintage People know when to jump rather than to just sit and get burned. That is a very valuable skill.

Vintage People have learned that they cannot please everyone. To be that flexible destroys the individual—and it is also impossible. In one of Aesop's fables he says, "Please all and you please none." Rev. Billy Graham puts it a little stronger when he writes, "The most prominent place in hell is reserved for those who are neutral on the great issues of life." And finally, Margaret Thatcher remarks, "Standing in the middle of the road is very dangerous; you get knocked down by the traffic from both sides!" What a great skill we can glean from the Vintage People who have invested their lives maturing and arriving at a point where they can be flexible in appropriate matters but still stand firm in the progress of mankind. It is a noble goal.

SEVEN

ACTION

"To live is not merely to breathe: it is to act;
it is to make
use of our organs, senses, faculties—of all
those parts
of ourselves which give us the feeling of
existence."
—Jean Jacques Rousseau

V intage People are people of action. In my first job at a gas station and car wash my boss, a very Vintage Person, had a favorite saying that he teased me with over and over. If a piece of equipment broke or a situation arose, and I didn't know what to do, he would say, "Well, do something, even if it is wrong!"

I think that turned out to be pretty good advice. We now know that people of action are much better adjusted and are happier people. They suffer less depression. Modern theories of psychiatry suggest that action is the one thing in our lives that we do have control over. We can't always control our circumstances; we can't always control how we feel; but we can control the action we take in any situation. Oliver Wendell Holmes said, "Life is action!"

There is something about action that is ingrained in the human spirit. Consider, for example, the people Jesus healed. Each healing required some action from the person being healed. Doctor Luke, a physician, describes even the

simple action of touching the hem of Jesus' garment healing the lady with years of menstrual bleeding. "Go and
wash," Jesus told the blind man. "Stretch out your hand,"
He told the leper. "Throw down your crutches," He told the
lame. Each required some action. I think it is significant
that Jesus never just walked up to someone with an afflic-
tion and healed them. They had to ask, and they all had to
perform some action. There is something about action and
the human spirit that makes people feel better. It helps with
healing and with keeping us healthy.

Let me illustrate what a big factor action is in the way
humans feel. The history of medicine is full of stories of
quackery. Successful quackery involves the patient taking
some sort of action that changes the way he feels. One of
the most bizarre examples of this took place around the
beginning of the twentieth century right here in southern
Kansas.

A practitioner by the name of Dr. John Romulus Brinkley came to Kansas in 1916 and attracted a national following by performance of "goat gland" transplants, which
were advertised as being able to restore masculine virility.
When doing these surgeries became too much work he
developed a "cure" for aches, pains, fatigue, arthritis, and
whatever other symptoms one might have. His therapy con-
sisted of a black box with a lot of knobs and lights. Initially
the patients were required to come to his office and sit in a
special chair. The electrodes were hooked up to them, and
he "cleansed" their bodies for twenty minutes. The patients
paid a good sum for therapy, and they did feel better!

Dr. Brinkley was so successful that soon there were
not enough twenty-minute slots per day for all his patients
wanting therapy. His creativity solved this dilemma. He
decided that through the miracles of modern technology
he didn't even need the patients to come into his office. He

could "beam" treatments out to them in their own homes. Again, action would be required. Each patient was assigned a specific time to go sit in a comfortable chair, in their own living room, for twenty minutes on their appointed days. He could then beam out the treatments to an endless number of patients at the same time. The only other thing required was for the patients to mail in their payments regularly!

Sounds absurd doesn't it? But this happened less than one hundred years ago. At one time Dr. Brinkley was so popular that he ran for governor in the state of Kansas. Finally the medical societies found that he had no formal medical training and exerted enough pressure that the good doctor moved to Texas for a while. He built a big practice there as well. Again pressure mounted, and he finally had to move across the Mexican border where he continued to beam his treatments across to his patients in Texas. And they kept sending in their money!

The human mind interprets certain actions as important to how we feel. Whether it is a treatment beamed to us at certain times, exercise, good nutrition, or a sense of accomplishment, action is imperative in fulfilling our expectations.

Use it or lose it

Writing in the fifth century B.C., Hippocrates made the following observation: "All parts of the body which have function, if used in moderation and exercised in labors to which each is accustomed, become thereby well developed and age slowly, but if unused and left idle, they become liable to disease, defective in growth and age quickly."

Stated in modern language this is the "Use it or lose it" principle. Vintage People have discovered this medical

fact. Practically all of the Vintage People I interviewed
held to this concept of bodily exercise—and mental exercise as well. Many stated it exactly that way—"use it or
lose it." This is a general physiological principle in medicine. It applies to all muscles and glands and to the brain as
well.

Physical exercise

When speaking of physical exercise, Guy, an eighty-year-
old Vintage Gentleman, told me, "I figure if I don't do
something today, I sure won't be able to do it tomorrow!"

I will never forget the delightful eighty-eight-year-old
woman I treated for sore knees. Her knees were red and
inflamed. "What have you been doing?" I asked her.

"I've taken up clogging," she explained. "I just love the
dancing, and my group just won a contest!"

"Dancing in wooden shoes is not the best thing for your
arthritic knees," I told her.

"Oh, I know that," she replied. "But I would just as
soon wear out these old knees than to have them rust out!"

Science has confirmed what these people have discovered for themselves. Statistics show that most elderly people who become physically dependent die within one year.
In the past, we felt that disease was the cause of the inactivity. But we are now learning that dependency or inactivity can cause disease. Much of what we once considered as
simple aging may actually be changes that occur secondary to disuse. Grace A. Cordts, M.D., states, "There are
striking similarities between structural and functional
declines associated with aging and the effects of enforced
inactivity."

Most of the time the goal of exercise for Vintage People
is not to be competitive in some sport or to build a "Mr. or

Miss Universe" body. The goal is to feel good, to have fun, and to be proficient at performing activities of daily living. Extremely vigorous exercise is not needed. Most medical authorities now agree that good physical fitness requires only twenty minutes of quickened heart rate three times a week. By a quickened heart rate, I mean exercising to maintain your pulse rate at 60 to 80 percent of its maximum for twenty minutes. Pardon the scientific talk, but an easy way to figure maximum heart rate for your age is to subtract your age, in years, from the number 220. So the formula is 220 minus age, times 60 to 80 percent. Books and exercise programs are available that explain all kinds of aerobic programs.

Doctors don't all agree on how much medical testing is necessary before someone starts an exercise program. Some feel that to be safe, a complete physical exam, blood work, and stress or treadmill EKG are needed. Others feel that exercise is a normal part of life, and therefore no special screening is needed for normal healthy individuals. I personally like the approach of the Royal College of Physicians and British Cardiology Society. They basically feel that no medical exam is necessary, in people with no symptoms as long as the exercise program starts at a low level and then progressively builds. This is the "common sense" approach. Anyone with symptoms or with a history of serious illness such as heart attacks, heart failure, or other medical problems, needs to see his physician who is acquainted with his or her limitations. Also, anyone who is planning to take up a vigorous exercise program or training for a competitive sport should seek the advice of a personal physician.

Not only the elderly suffer from the lack of activity. Just over 50 years ago, obstetricians routinely kept their new mothers at bed rest for ten days after delivery. They were trying to prevent complications from childbirth, such as blood clots and infection. The incidence of blood clots in the legs—or "milk leg" as it was known then—was high. We now know that one of the main causes of blood clots in the legs is inactivity! Doctors were causing the disease they were trying to prevent! Once we began getting new mothers up and about soon after delivery, this complication became less frequent and now has all but gone away.

A number of studies show that people who exercise regularly or stay physically active by whatever means at any age require less medical treatment and less institutionalization than non-exercisers. Notice that I said, "at any age." This implies that we cannot just wait until we are approaching advanced years to start exercising. I don't want to beat this to death, but I have had too many patients tell me that they plan to start walking, or start riding their bicycles, or play more golf, or tennis, or whatever—after they retire. After all, they will have time to do this after retirement. I've also been called to the hospital to see these people for their heart attacks a week after they retire!

An athletic Vintage Patient of mine who walks at a local middle school track every morning explained to me, "I've seen people show up at the track after retirement, or after something like a heart attack. They start out all bent over and out of breath. They can't even walk a block at first. But if they stick with it, in a month or so they really start to step out! They get up to two to four miles in no time. But I've seen some try it and drop out. I just watch the paper and pretty soon I see their names in the obits!"

Almost all the Vintage People that I interviewed had a healthy life-style in middle age as well as in their Vintage Years. They entered their Vintage Years in good physical shape. One of my oldest patients, who was able to live independently until the very end, recently died at the age of

108. She was a retired high school physical education teacher and continued to do calisthenics every morning and to take daily walks. She had been active all her life, and attributed her longevity to exercise. Vintage People also realize that exercise needs to be consistent to be effective. One of the things I have observed in my medical career, but don't really like to admit to myself, is how fast exercise wears off. Without exercise the body deteriorates much more rapidly than any of us would like. Talk to the athlete in training who by missing just a few days notices a big decrease in his or her performance. I've taken care of a number of ex-high school and college athletes who are in great physical shape when they graduate. Then they give up their sport, go to work and develop a sedentary life-style. On their next yearly physical exam, the benefits of years of physical activity and training have been erased. They have gained weight, their pulse and blood pressure is up, and their endurance for stress is down. It doesn't seem fair, but the body requires frequent exercise to maintain itself.

One of the serious problems physicians dealing with space medicine are encountering in space travel is rapid deconditioning of the body in space due to the lack of gravity. Here on earth we get a certain amount of exercise by just rolling over, standing up or walking. In space you simply float everywhere effortlessly. Even relatively short missions of a few weeks in space bring devastating effects. Prior to the development of exercise programs for space, the astronauts often had to be carried off the space shuttle because they had become too weak to walk. On today's space stations astronauts are secured to a treadmill by large rubber bands that simulate gravity. They must walk or run on the treadmill approximately six hours a day to maintain their physical strength.

Recent studies show that even the sedentary, frail elderly can benefit from a physical therapy program aimed at slowly increasing physical activity. It has been shown that, with proper exercise, even nursing home residents in their nineties can improve such things as functional capacity, balance, grip strength, and self-ratings of depression. Weight lifting seems to be particularly good in building muscle tone. Even bedridden individuals who are given simple range of motion exercises have fewer contractures and are better able to facilitate the tasks of their caregivers. That is good news to those of us who are still active and who hope to become Vintage People some day.

It is never too late to start exercising. But what exercise is best? Do we all have to take up jogging in order to be healthy? I don't think so! To me exercise is physiological, a part of living. If we look back only a few centuries, exercise was indeed a part of everyday life. Everyone had to walk wherever he went. Obtaining food required exercise, not only in catching or harvesting it, but also in rather lengthy preparation. Physical work was a way of life. The body was kept in tone almost naturally in order for the individual to survive.

Watch children at play. They exercise! They don't have to think about it or plan it. They don't need expensive exercise equipment. They don't need to dress in tights and drive to classes at a gym across town. They don't care if they have $200 running shoes or spandex! To them, exercise is natural—a part of everyday life. And they have FUN. And to me that is the most important part of exercise. If it is not fun, you are not going to do it. Children at play are an excellent example to us adults as to what exercise should be. It has to be enjoyable.

In addition to having fun, children naturally limit themselves. This is another valuable lesson for adults. Kids don't abuse their bodies like adults do. I don't see overexertion injuries in children—until adults get involved. Kids can play baseball on the vacant lot in the neighborhood without any equipment in all the broken glass, gopher holes, and thorn bushes, and never get hurt. Adults come along and provide them with a perfectly smooth, fenced, clean baseball field, cleats, batting helmets, and catchers mitts. And then what happens? We begin to see knee injuries, broken ankles and all kinds of overuse syndromes. What has happened? The adults are now pushing the kids in their exercise potential. They no longer are playing just for fun. They don't or can't stop and go home when they get tired like they did before. They have to try harder to please the adults.

And herein is my point about exercise. Stop when you are tired. Most of us are not training for a marathon. Nor do we need to be able to run a marathon in order to be healthy. If achieving a healthy body with increased energy and improved capacity for unexpected demands is our goal, exercise needs to be fun. We don't need to push. The common phrase, "No pain, no gain," only applies to exercise for persons who are actively training for some specific goal. If you just want to be healthy, walk until you are tired and quit!

One of the best axioms concerning exercise came from one of my professors in medical school. He said, "The human body was not built to run long distances. Humans were designed to run real fast for short distances, climb a tree, and then sit there and use their brain to figure out a way of escape!"

What kinds of exercise do most Vintage People do? Surprisingly, one of the favorite forms of "exercise" that I found in the people interviewed was doing work or performing tasks of some kind. Housework was popular among the ladies. Yard-work or woodworking was popular for the men. One ninety-two-year-old explained it well: "When I putter in my workshop I get exercise, but I'm also able to combine that with a sense of accomplishing something at the same time. Both of those things help me feel better!"

The next most popular form of exercise is walking, one of the best and most physiologic forms of exercise. It is cheap, involves almost all the muscles of the body and gives the heart and lungs a good workout. Overexertion or injury is seldom seen with walking. All the Vintage People that I interviewed recommended walking—even though some were no longer able to perform this function.

Swimming, bowling, bicycling, and even jogging are enjoyed by some of the Vintage People I know. Interestingly, the common key to all their various forms of exercise, is that they are doing something they enjoy. They are having fun, the most important feature of physical fitness that Vintage People have discovered. The rest of us need to remember this. Too many of us rush into a vigorous, strenuous exercise program that is no fun. We soon burn out. The right kind of exercise is fun! We need to return the fun to it.

It is my practice to ask my patients about exercise and their activity level at each office visit. "Are you getting any exercise? What do you do to stay active?" It gives me a very important clue to their general health status. I think asking these questions helps motivate them to remain active. I have probably prevented more disease by encouraging my patients to be active than by any other single thing that I have done as a physician. An "exercise prescription" written specifically for each patient has probably saved more lives than open heart surgery, organ transplants and all forms of cardiopulmonary resuscitation combined. Exercise is an important form of therapy and good health.

Lack of physical exercise and activity however, is not always just laziness or a life-style choice. Often it is forced upon us. I know Vintage People, who for a number of medical reasons, are not able to do much physical exercise. One man I know is now paralyzed from the neck down from a neurological disease. Concerning exercise, he states: "I always felt better when I exercised. I did as much as I could until my disease robbed me of that function. For a while I could only raise my arms and wave them about. Now I can only exercise my neck muscles, but I do that every day."

One of my medical school professors told me one time that "no one ever dies from arthritis." He was wrong! (Actually, about fifty percent of what I learned in medical school has turned out to be wrong according to today's beliefs!) If the pain and stiffness of arthritis leads to forced inactivity, which I have seen it do, the other systems of the body also begin to suffer. Muscles deteriorate from the lack of walking. Patients may gain weight, which makes them more prone to such diseases as diabetes and further degenerative arthritis. With lack of exercise, the heart and lungs begin to suffer. If the heart is weak, it does not pump sufficient blood to the kidneys, and renal failure sets in. With kidney disease comes a higher incidence of high blood pressure, which can lead to strokes and heart attacks. This is known as the "cascade effect" in geriatric medicine. I think that term accurately describes the doomed pathway that inactivity brings.

We must not forget that the body functions as a whole. We cannot ignore any part of it. Inability or disability in one system often leads to difficulties in another system unless there is some compensation. Exercise can interrupt the cascade effect. Proper exercise has been shown to increase total physical well-being and general health by improving cardiorespiratory capacity, muscle strength, flexibility, resistance to disease, sleep and even cognitive function. Some form of physical therapy or exercise is used in almost all diseases afflicting people of all ages. Range of motion exercises can be done on the most seriously ill patients—even those on life support in the intensive care unit—and it has been shown to be beneficial.

Mental exercise

The "use it or lose it" principle of medicine also applies to the brain. Actually, this is probably the major application. My patient with multiple sclerosis explains, "I can't use my legs, I can't use my arms, but I can still keep my mind sharp. I've learned that mental exercise is essential."

My Vintage Patients who continue to learn stay sharp mentally. This makes sense. Several years ago there was a public awareness push about "Infant Stimulation." Simply put, research showed that babies exposed to a lot of stimulation, such as contrasting colors, mobiles, touch, holding, being talked to, and played with develop their brains at a faster pace than those who receive less stimulation. This applies not only to babies but to all of us throughout our lives.

Of all the parts of our body, the brain has the greatest capacity for stretching and growing. You can build your biceps only to a certain level, and you can run only so fast, but your brain's capacity is virtually limitless. The highest estimate of brain function that Margaret Mead, the world recognized American anthropologist, makes is ten percent efficiency. The potential is tremendous. As a matter of fact, the more you learn, the more your ability to learn increases. With the advent of the computer we have a model to explain some of the workings of the brain. As I heard a speaker at a medical seminar say one time, "Our brains are like a computer—made of meat!" The more information that is fed in the more potential connections that can be made. Research shows that we can increase our IQ by increasing our vocabulary.

I have witnessed the fantastic ability of the brain to learn while caring for patients with strokes. It takes more work than an infant seems to put into it, but patients can re-learn many things as new pathways are created within the brain. Imagine learning to talk again at the age of eighty-eight after a stroke, or learning to walk again at that age. It is difficult, but I have a patient in the hospital right now who has accomplished just that. I call it persistence and determination; his family calls it just plain stubbornness. But whatever it is, this Vintage Person is stretching his brain and has accomplished far more than any of his physicians and physical therapists thought possible.

New experiences are the best way to keep the brain alert. New ways of thinking are especially effective. Vintage People like to expose themselves to new things. Learning a foreign language or beginning a musical instrument seems to be especially stimulating. Research indicates that these activities tap neurons in the brain that haven't been previously used. Hence, more neuroconnections can be made, and the brain has more information to work with. Thus there is almost a chain reaction. The more we learn, the more capacity we have to learn.

Just like physical exercise, mental exercise should also be fun. If it is not fun, it is only human nature to avoid it. I recently was invited to address a college class called "This and That." It is made up exclusively of people in their seventies, eighties, and a few in their nineties. They earn college credit while hearing various people lecture about an assortment of topics—an effective way to keep the mind young. My Toastmasters Club has several Vintage Members who are keeping their minds in shape with public speaking, and they are having fun at the same time.

Here, as in all aspects of their lives, Vintage People tend to be creative. One lady I know stimulates herself mentally by working puzzles of increasing difficulty. Reading is common; so is listening to tapes—especially for those with eyesight problems. An eighty-four-year-old retired piano teacher in my practice who recently suffered a mild stroke, has just set out to learn all the works of Mozart. Following the stroke, she had been confused mentally and had trouble controlling her right hand. She explained to me, "I had to do something to blow the cobwebs out of my brain!" It is working. She is much more alert on each office visit, and is now sharper mentally than many of my younger patients! As amazing as it may seem, she has re-learned much of the coordination that she once had in the right hand. Her piano playing is coming along remarkably well.

There is also evidence that vigorous physical exercise can help keep the brain in shape. In one study, going for a walk was compared to eating a candy bar or taking a one-hour nap before taking a standardized written test. Those who had just gone for a walk repeatedly did better on the exam. Even after the roles were changed, those who exercised performed better on the exam. As one vigorous eighty-eight-year-old Vintage Gentleman observes: "I know I often get some of my best ideas while walking or jogging. And I have noticed that my mind remains sharper for several hours after such an exercise. Walking or jogging is much more refreshing and invigorating for me than taking a nap!"

People tend to think that exercise will leave them more tired than when they started. In truth, exercise will make you less tired mentally and physically. I have trouble trying to convince my patients of that. But try it, and I know you will find it to be true.

On the other hand, watching TV seems to require about the same amount of brain energy as staring at a wall or watching paint dry. Laboratory studies with brain imaging have repeatedly shown this. Television isn't all bad. It just depends upon what you are watching and for how long. However, if you are watching TV, you can't be doing something else. A patient once asked me, "Did you ever wonder why the people we watch on TV never watch TV? It's because if they spent their time watching TV, their lives would be too dull for us to watch!"

When I ask my Vintage Patients what they watch on TV, two main answers come up. The number one answer is "The news!" The other is the "Discovery Channel." When I visit patients in the nursing home, they are usually propped up around a big screen watching soap operas, game shows, or talk shows. These may be entertaining, but—in my opinion—have very little to do with keeping the brain sharp.

Finally, Vintage People have learned how to keep their brains optimistic. Science is still struggling to learn more about this phenomenon, but we do know that positive signals can actually change the structure of the perception process. The late, great Dr. Norman Vincent Peale spent his lifetime writing and lecturing on this subject. By changing your attitude and looking for the good in any situation, you can actually create positive circuitry in the brain that changes the way you respond, and the way you feel. You will actually see challenges instead of threats or despair in difficult situations. As Dr. Peale states, there is definitely "Power" in positive thinking! And science is beginning to agree with this concept, although we still cannot explain it. The optimistic attitude will be mentioned over and over, as I have found it to be a major characteristic of Vintage People.

Hard work

Vintage People are never lazy. Osborn Segerberg Jr. surveyed 1,200 centenarians and reported that "hard work" was the most frequently given reason for living so long. In my own interaction with my patients I find that to be true, but with an interesting twist—not only that they have worked hard all their lives, but that they *enjoyed* working. I have found few "workaholics" in this group, if you define a workaholic as a compulsive neurotic who works non-stop without pleasure. Vintage People may put in a lot of hours, but they enjoy what they are doing. As Confucius said, "If you love what you do, you will never work another day in your life!"

Several years ago I had an eighty-four-year-old patient who owned and operated a lumberyard. This Vintage Man continued to work five and a half days a week. He took care of more customers than the other half dozen employees put together because he knew his products and knew where everything was located. Customers requested him because of his practical knowledge. He waited on me one day just two weeks after I had helped with his hernia repair—a condition he had developed from the hard work of loading and unloading lumber for his customers. I asked him why he was back at work so soon after surgery. After all, that type of operation frequently kept younger guys from doing heavy manual labor for at least six weeks. I suggested that he might at least want to be on the golf course, or perhaps fishing. His reply helped me understand his longevity and good health. He replied, "Doc, there's just no other place I would rather be than right here! This is not work to me! Work is doing something you don't want to do!" He would rather be there in his lumberyard helping his customers than anywhere else in this world. He is a man of action, who enjoys what he is doing. George Burns described it well when he said: "Fall in love with what you are going to do for a living. To be able to get out of bed and do what you love to do for the rest of the day is beyond words."

The benefits of work are not all physical. Researchers have found that people in their seventies who continued to work "strenuously" maintained their mental sharpness better than those who were not involved in a work situation. Of course, many of these characteristics like mental "sharpness" are very hard to measure and compare scientifically. But I've seen it over and over in my patients. I don't need to put a number on it to know that it is true.

One might argue that the reason Vintage People continue to work is because they remain healthier and sharper mentally. It makes sense that people who are healthy, who feel good, and remain mentally sharp are better able to work. Their minds demand the stimulation that work provides. This is like the old question, which comes first, the chicken or the egg? Does hard work create Vintage People, or do Vintage People simply look for work to do?

My answer to this question is—both! In all other aspects of life, one first has to have some talent, motivation or characteristic to develop. Hard work is used to develop those talents. As one talent is developed, other talents begin to surface. The motivation for hard work seems to be the "stuff" that success is made of.

Let's take athletics for example. To be a good athlete, one has to have some natural athletic skills or talents. Next, motivation is essential. Then with hard work, the athlete begins to see what his or her potential is. Other doors begin to open as his talents and skills develop. But it is the hard work that keeps him competitive. Athletic abilities alone might help the backyard athlete, but anyone who wishes to be competitive knows that hard work and training is going to be involved. Any athlete can tell you how quickly he will lose his sharpness if he stops training—that is, if he stops the hard work that keeps him where he is.

It is also that way in business, in politics, in academics. Those who rise to the top have some natural talent, but they also combine it with hard work that tempers the talents and keeps the cutting edge sharp! There is no reason to believe it is any different with aging. Most Vintage People have been relatively successful in earlier life. The hard work and continued training seems to be the honing stone that keeps their cutting edge sharp and prevents rust and corrosion from setting in. This gets back to the principle of "use it or lose it." Better to wear out than rust out!

The final convincing argument for the benefits of hard work is what Vintage People themselves say. In interview after interview, Vintage People mention hard work as one of the primary factors that has kept them healthy and productive. Many Vintage People I interviewed were quick to point out the rewards of hard work. Something about accomplishment makes one feel worthwhile and needed. One eighty-year-old explained: "My younger friends are always saying that I work so hard just to keep busy—for something to do. That makes me so mad! I don't stay busy *for something to do*, I stay busy *to do something!*"

Accomplishment

Vintage People are motivated people. They love the sense of accomplishment. They thrive on it. As a matter of fact, their day doesn't seem complete unless they have accomplished some feat—large or small. An eighty-one-year-old nurse says, "I do something every day that makes me feel as though I've accomplished something, even if it's only making a batch of jelly." Another states, "I am a person who must contribute something every day, and feel incomplete if I do not."

I've often wondered why some people are self-motivated and others are not. Neurochemists are trying to explain motivation now on the basis of certain neurotransmitters in the brain. I visited with a pharmaceutical salesman in my office recently who claimed that the new antidepressant medication that he was selling could affect motivation. It's a vague claim at present, but by changing the chemicals in the brain, he felt that those who take this medication will feel less depressed and also be more motivated. Wouldn't that be a great medication! It should go into the public water supply!

Of course, motivation is hard to measure. There is no "motivation meter" and no blood test for it. Maybe it is chemical, as the salesman is suggesting. Perhaps it is genetic, like blue eyes. Perhaps it has to do with environment and one's surroundings. Perhaps it's a characteristic that we learn in childhood from our parents. Or maybe it is just one of those qualities that dwells deep in the human spirit that we will never understand—a gift.

I am, however, convinced that the pharmaceutical salesman was right about one thing. Human motivation can be changed. I'm not convinced yet that his pills will do it, but it does happen. I don't think it is all physical. When I've seen it happen, it is usually something that touches the mind. Most of the people that I have seen go from no motivation to being a very motivated person have done so because of words, thoughts, or ideas. We see this in religion when someone suddenly "sees the light" and becomes motivated. Large corporations spend huge sums of money on motivational seminars for their employees—and it sometimes works! Dr. Norman Vincent Peale says we can become motivated towards accomplishment by the following process: "Plant the seeds of expectation in your mind; cultivate thoughts that anticipate achievement. Believe in yourself as being capable of overcoming all obstacles and weaknesses."

Motivation is not something we can give to someone. A lot of things help, but the spark still has to come from within the person. And if you have it, you are on your way to becoming a Vintage Person. Vintage People feel a thrill of accomplishment. They are people of action who are motivated to seek out this thrill of achievement through hard work and activity.

Dr. Martin Luther King, Jr., described a Vintage Person very well when he said, "If you are called to be a street sweeper, sweep streets even as Michelangelo painted, or Beethoven composed music, or Shakespeare wrote poetry. Sweep streets so well that all the hosts of heaven and earth will pause to say, here lived a great street sweeper who did his job well."

Serving others

A number of Vintage People have found service to be the key to their happiness. As Albert Schweitzer said, "...the only ones among you who will be really happy are those who have sought and found how to serve." Dr. Martin Luther King Jr. said it this way, "Everybody can be great, because anybody can serve. You don't have to have a college degree to serve. You don't have to make your subject and verb agree to serve....You only need a heart full of grace, a soul generated by love." There is power in serving. As people age, their goals become less material and more altruistic. The joy received from volunteer work in the hospital, in pubic service organizations, in churches, and even in business becomes more important. Suddenly the money seems less important than the service itself. I think Vintage People begin to realize that satisfaction really does come from helping others.

For a long time therapists have encouraged depressed patients to find someone to help. The mere act of helping someone else, taking action, helps the depressed patient feel better. I often use this suggestion in therapy when patients become depressed or obsessed with their own illness and problems. Something about helping others helps us forget ourselves. This has been known since antiquity, and many religions have incorporated service to others into their instructions for living.

Several years ago I had a negative, miserable patient who was driving me crazy. Doctors know the type all too well. This woman's children were grown and living in other cities with families and concerns of their own. She had stopped venturing out except for her frequent doctor's appointments and had turned all of her worries and energies inward. On every office visit she brought a long list of complaints, most of which had very little physical basis. She never followed instructions, and nothing I did for her ever helped. She read everything she could about all the dread diseases of mankind and was convinced that she had every one of them.

I knew the pattern. She was withdrawn and depressed. But nothing I was able to do could persuade her of that diagnosis. We had tried several anti-depressant medications, but she always seemed to have some minor side effects and stopped them a few days before they'd had time to take effect. I suspected she didn't really want to be any better, both because she was enjoying her own misery and because the doctor's appointments were her social contact. If she got better, I might not have her come in as often.

Needless to say, my office staff and I were getting desperate. Several other doctors in town had already refused to see her. Finally I decided to challenge her. I knew if I could get her mind off herself, and onto something or someone else, it would help her life and her health. We had to pull her out of the mess of pessimistic self-pity that she was wallowing in.

One afternoon before she could even start on her list, I looked her straight in the eye, and said with enthusiasm, "Gladys, I've just gotten back from a Family Practice convention where I went to a seminar about people that have problems just like yours." She raised her eyebrows but continued to listen.

"Now, you are probably going to think this is stupid, but I know it will work for you, and I'm excited for you to try it! You know we have done every test in the book, and those have all turned out good. But the one thing we can't test is what I think is causing you to feel so bad. I think your brain chemistry is low. Doctors have learned that when people are stimulated and motivated, there are more of these certain chemicals in the brain, kind of like adrenaline to your body. We know that when babies are not stimulated properly, they don't develop normally. We also know that a violin string when it's too loose and not stressed a little can't make beautiful music. Your brain is like that, and I think it's causing all the problems that you have on your list."

I was surprised, but she was still listening, so I continued. "Gladys, I want to try a program on you that I learned about at that seminar. I want to set you up in a volunteer program to help at one of the nursing homes here in town. My nurse will make all the arrangements, so all you have to do is show up once a week for four hours. You will see people there who have worse health and more problems than you do. You can help these people. More than that, I promise you that if you will try this for three weeks, you will feel better yourself!"

Before she could respond, I got up and left the room. My nurse called the nursing home and explained the situation. They even agreed to provide transportation for Gladys and said they would pick her up at home the next day.

I was trying to avoid her as she left the exam room for fear that she would have multiple reasons why she could not do this and turn the idea down flat. But when she passed me in the hall, she stopped, looked over the top of her glasses, folded up her list of complaints and said, "Well, if I try this, I'm only doing it to show you how wrong you are!"

I knew I had gone out on a limb, but I was looking forward to her next appointment so I could find out if this had worked. I was disappointed when she again unfolded her list and said, "Doc, you are wrong! Working out there made my arthritis flare up. I was so tired I could hardly move when I got home. I'm having more headaches and my feet hurt! I think this is a stupid idea! Besides, there is no one out there that is worse off than me!"

To my total surprise, when she was leaving, she commented, "I guess I better get home and rest up, since I have to do that volunteer work tomorrow!" She kept her commitment to go ahead and volunteer for two more weeks as we had originally agreed.

I was dreading her return appointment at the end of the third week. To my astonishment she canceled her appointment at the last minute and didn't show up. This had never happened before. Going to the doctor was the highlight of her life. I had my nurse call to be sure everything was all right. All afternoon we were unable to reach her. Finally about 6 p.m. she answered the phone. "Oh no, nothing is wrong," she replied. "We were having a birthday party for Mrs. Foster today, and I just couldn't miss it! She turned 100 years old today, you know!"

She never did admit to me the changes that had taken place in her life, but she didn't make another doctor's appointment for over six months, and that was for an ankle sprain she had sustained while at a dance!

If this doesn't show the power of action and serving others, I don't know what would. When people are serving, life has meaning.

EIGHT

HEALTH AND MEDICINE

"O health! health! the blessing of the rich! the riches
of the poor! who can buy thee at too dear a rate,
since there is no enjoying this world
without thee?"

—Ben Jonson

Konrad Adenauer was still chancellor of West Germany at the age of eighty. He was complaining to his physician about his slow recovery from the flu. To this his physician responded, "I'm not a magician! I can't make you young again!"

Adenauer, who was anxious to get back to work replied, "I'm not asking that! I don't want to become young again. All I want is to go on getting older!"

In our society anyone who lives to a Vintage Age will have most likely encountered the medical profession along the way. A large percentage of the medical services performed in this country are for people over sixty-five. I was surprised that the Vintage People I interviewed were selective in their "doctoring." Most had previously had some significant illnesses, but once they were well, they avoided excessive medical treatments and medications.

Even so, health is one of the major concerns of all the Vintage People I interviewed. They are aware of their health and their limitations. They are careful in their dealings with the medical profession, and equally careful with medications and nutrition.

The medical profession is getting better at understanding Vintage People. Attitudes of patients and physicians alike have changed, and people today generally accept the reality that age is no longer a measurement of years but a measurement of function.

The medical profession

The first textbook of geriatric medicine that I ever owned is still on my bookshelf. It was published in 1978 and was the first book I had found that was devoted entirely to the subject of medical care of older patients. How our concepts have changed! This textbook has a black and white photo on the cover of a cute, frail, "little old lady" sitting in a wheelchair. Her hair is thin and white. Her skin is wrinkled, and she is wearing a sweater with a handkerchief partially showing from one of the sleeves. She has cute, little, round, thick glasses. She is wearing no jewelry or make-up. The wall behind her is blank, and it appears that she probably lives in some type of institution.

This woman's doctor has been kind enough to come to visit her, as it is implied in the photo that she certainly could not get out. The kindly doctor, complete in coat and tie as well as plaid pants, is bending down to his patient. And to show her gratitude, the little old lady is gripping his hand with hers, and holding it to her cheek, with a broad smile on her face.

As I sat looking at this now, I thought, what stereotyping! What a prejudiced view of aging! And this was from the medical profession? I know it was not intentional and that it reflected the feelings of society about aging at that time, but aren't physicians supposed to be aware of such typecasting? How could we have missed the mark so far? It makes me wonder what else we are missing now as authority figures to many of our patients. If this is what physicians expect of old age, won't the public expect the same thing? After all, the doctor should know about aging. What we expect to happen gets set in our minds, and it often becomes reality simply because we believe it to be so.

Physicians didn't understand aging at that time. We were treating aging as a disease—something to be prevented or cured. We were taught to be kind, understanding, and compassionate to the "old people," but medicine pretty much ignored the special problems of this group. We may even have made things worse. We treated older people with the same medications and remedies we used on our younger patients. We encouraged nursing home placement where grandma or grandpa could be "taken care of" and therefore maintain his or her physical health. Society blessed this approach to medical care.

Such an approach to aging is dangerous! The human body changes as we age. We would not think of giving a baby or a child the same medications and the same doses as we give an adult. Yet we often did that to the older patient. The most common problem is that as we age, our metabolism slows down. If you don't think so, try to eat the way you did when you were a teenager and see what happens! The percentage of the body that is muscle mass, fat, and water, all change. The functions of the liver and kidneys slow down. Those two organs eliminate about ninety percent of all medications from the body. You can begin to see how medications may build up in the older person, and that they can literally be overdosed on an amount of medication that would be appropriate for a younger individual. Exercise requirements change. Nutritional requirements change.

Our physical reserves decrease remarkably as we age. In youth, many organ systems such as the liver, lungs, and kidneys have a reserve capacity of about four times. Smoking, alcohol and other abuse factors, as well as diseases chip away at those reserves over the years. Once we get to that last one-fourth of the reserves of a vital organ, any more decrease causes a big difference. This is a little like flying in a four-engine airplane. With one engine out, it can still fly fairly well; two engines out and it slows down; three engines out, and it can barely stay in the air; but when the fourth engine goes, it's all over! In geriatric medicine, preserving that last engine is important. Here more that anywhere else, an ounce of prevention is worth a pound of cure.

Just as children are not physiologically "little adults," older patients are not medically "old adults." Age is not a disease. Normal changes take place in metabolism and in physical reserves. The physician who does not recognize this fact will often overdose his or her older patients, causing organ damage, somnolence, low blood pressure, unnecessary sedation, confusion and a host of other medical and social problems.

What about the idea of placing older people into institutions to protect their health? When I think of this, I reflect back to my Kansas farm background. My father raised hogs. We fed them daily, but since they were free out in the fields they also did a lot of foraging for themselves. They rooted for insects in the soil and ate tender green grass, weeds or leaves—whatever nature provided. In the heat of summer they wallowed in the mud. In season, we fed them left-over apples, sweet corn, and other garden produce. As they lay under the shade of a big oak tree eating farm grown corn, I could even imagine a smile on their faces. Life was good! Of course, they eventually went to market, but I always justified that by believing that they had a quality life while they were on the farm.

A few years ago, I visited a modern hog farm. What a contrast! The certified baby pigs were born in a sterile environment by C-section to prevent any contamination. They were raised entirely inside a building that was heated in the winter and air-conditioned in the summer. They never saw dirt or the outdoors. They ate a scientifically prepared diet with all the proper vitamins and minerals but never tasted fresh produce. They never lay on the hillside in the sun or played in the mud. Physiologically, they did well and gained weight rapidly. Ultimately, they went to market. But after visiting this modern hog farm, I wondered which animals—those on the farm or those in the institutional setup—had any quality of life.

It seems to me that there is some comparison here with humans. In institutions such as nursing homes, a person can get all the care he or she needs to do well physically. But at what cost? How much quality is sacrificed? Is this controlled, sterile environment really living? I realize the time comes when reality demands convalescent care. I'm not saying we should never take care of the physical needs of our population. I do think we need to think about the trade-off. I have asked hundreds of patients about nursing home care and whether or not they want it. The answer is almost always the same. No! Many even qualify the statement by saying, "I would rather go home and die!"

Do we listen to these people? Somehow we feel that older people no longer have the right to make their own decisions. They are like children in that sense. Often they are forced into accepting the decisions their families make for them. They have no way to fight back. Even the right to handle their own financial affairs can be taken away by the courts. Our society says that preservation of physical well-being takes precedent over quality of life issues. Yet I admire the family member who is courageous enough to refuse a feeding tube or to give the permission to stop life support for an elderly relative.

Fortunately, there are now a few more options available. The trend is toward "assisted living" situations and apartments for the elderly. I've visited some very nice facilities in our area that provide the privacy of apartment living with the availability of prepared meals, nursing care when needed, and assistance in such things as bathing. Independence and quality of life are not totally destroyed.

In contrast to the picture of the "little old lady" on the front of my first textbook of geriatrics, the image is changing. Madison Avenue is frequently on the forefront of social change and reflects this in advertisements. Medical journals are not immune to this type of advertising. A recent ad for a heart medicine shows an older gentleman in full color. He is well tanned and wearing snorkel equipment while standing in the blue ocean with beautiful beaches and palm trees in the background. He has a beautiful smile and is holding his arms above his head as if in triumph. Children playing nearby look over at him as if in admiration. The caption reads, "Don't let Angina ruin one precious hour of your patient's day." What a wonderful new expectation we are setting for our Vintage Patients!

Medications

Vintage People take few medications. You may argue that if you are blessed with good health, few medications are required. I have a strong suspicion that the reverse is also true. Many times, the fewer medications you take, the healthier you are. Before everyone throws away their blood pressure pills, let me explain what I mean.

There is no question that medications such as insulin, antibiotics, immunizations, and antihypertensives, have vastly prolonged our life span and contributed to good health. However, as one of my professors in medical school pointed out, "Every medication is also a poison!" Every medication has side effects—the proverbial two-edged sword. All medications are foreign to the homeostasis of our body. It is imperative that they are used for the right things and in the proper amounts. Just because a medication does not require a prescription or a visit to the doctor does not mean it is not a potent chemical with possible bad side effects. Often patients tell me they are taking no medications when I am obtaining the medical history. If I ask them about what they take for their headache, they may be taking frequent aspirin, ibuprofen and other over-the-counter medications—all of which may be contributing to their ulcer condition. Antacids, vitamins, and preparations from the health food store are all medications as far as your body is concerned, and all are potential poisons.

Just because a compound is labeled "natural" does not mean it is good for you or without risks. Hemlock is natural, but it can kill you! Dirt is natural, but we shouldn't eat it. Believe me, after twenty years of medical practice, I have seen a lot of "natural" things lurking on the Kansas prairies that are not good for humans. The whole idea of "natural" vitamins and supplements is misleading. A vitamin C molecule, for example, doesn't know if it came from a "natural" source, or was brewed in the laboratory. The molecule is the same. Paying extra for something just because it is "natural" doesn't make sense—unless you are selling it!

Multiple medications or "poly-pharmacy" presents one of the most dangerous health problems for older people today. Many medications cross-react with one another. It is easy to think of taking one medication for your sinuses, another for cough, one for fever, and still another for blood pressure. Don't forget vitamin C for the cold, sleeping pills at night, and ginseng root from the health food store for energy. Medications can build up very quickly.

One of my attending physicians in medical school, whom I respect very much, kept a watchful eye on the medications we residents and interns used on our patients. He had a rule of thumb that I have always tried to follow. He said, "If you have a patient on more than five medications at once, you are just treating side effects!" But, surveys show that hospitalized patients routinely receive between seven and thirteen different medications during their stay. The typical nursing home patient is on fifteen! This is a problem! Some medications even compete with one another. Taking too many medications is like driving a car with one foot on the accelerator and the other foot on the brake.

Without going into a lot of boring scientific explanation, I will just summarize that most medications are metabolized, or broken down, by the body into other compounds. Some of these breakdown products can react with other breakdown products, or with other medications, forming chemicals in the body that you do not want! For a patient taking more that five different medications, the risk of cross reactions becomes huge. If you have ever studied probability or chances of winning the lottery, you know that with greater than five numbers or compounds, the possible combinations become enormous. This is especially true when each original medication may break down into several other compounds.

I admit that I have some patients on more than five medications, and probably more taking things I don't know about, but I try to keep people on as few medications as possible. Some of my greatest medical cures have come from simply stopping someone's unnecessary medications.

My partner and I had been in town a short while when one of the older physicians, who had been in practice for decades, unexpectedly died. Over the next few months many of his patients began coming to us, as the "new guys" in town. We discovered that our predecessor had maintained a unique medical practice. Each of his patients came to the office for their first visit with plastic bags full of pharmacy bottles of medications. Each one was taking an average of ten to twelve different medications! The record was one patient on twenty-two medicines! Imagine all the cross reactions that are possible with that number of pills!

You don't need cross reactions to have side effects. The commonest cause of treatable impotence in men is blood pressure medication. A common cause of fatigue is medication. A common cause of insomnia is medication. Mental confusion, low potassium, constipation, urinary difficulty, chronic cough, rashes, dizziness, stomach upset, headache, muscle cramps, and diarrhea are all common things I see that are caused by medications.

As explained above, the changes of aging hinder the elimination of many medications from the body. Even patients who have been on the same medications for years may become toxic from those medications as they age and their bodies change. Dosages have to be adjusted frequently in Vintage People.

It's easy for medications to accumulate. I see this most commonly in nursing homes. The nurse will call the doctor on call late one night and ask for a sleeping pill. The next night a different doctor may get a call for an antibiotic for the same patient. Then the family wants something for the patient's "nerves," and the family doctor prescribes that. When making rounds I wonder why Gertrude suddenly won't even wake up to eat! She is on sixteen different medications, including antacids, aspirin for her arthritis, a little

Pepto-Bismol for diarrhea, and three or four different laxatives. I usually have fun stopping most of her medications and watching her get better.

My advice to my patients and to all Vintage People is to know your medications and what they are for. Modern medications are wonderful if used properly. But know the common side effects. Especially if you see more that one doctor or specialist, always take your medications to your office visits, or at the very least, a detailed list of your medications. Include the milligram dosage and how you take them. And don't forget to include the over-the-counter medications as they may be just as important.

Always be honest about your medications. I often see a patient entering the hospital or nursing home, and on about the third day getting sicker. They brought all their medicines from home in the pharmacy bottles just like they should. Some of the medicines are labeled three times a day, some are daily, and others are four times a day. The hospital or nursing home gives the medications to the patient just as prescribed. At home the patient frequently forgot the daily dosage; she had stopped the four times a day medicine completely because it made her feel "funny," and she was taking the three times a day medicine at bedtime. When institutionalized, there is sudden forced compliance, and she is overdosed!

Medications have improved our quality of life and our longevity, but they must be used with care. Medical Board exams for Geriatric Medicine are multiple choice. I quickly learned that if one of the answers is "stop medication," that is always the correct answer. Successful Vintage People seem to have learned that lesson and avoid unnecessary medications. They may be ahead of the medical profession in that respect.

Placebo effect

The word "placebo" comes from Latin and means "I shall please." In medicine, a placebo is anything that works simply because the patient thinks it is going to work. The results are attributed to a person's expectations or beliefs rather than to cold hard facts. Much to the dismay of researchers, the placebo effect is high in humans. If a medication or type of therapy works only thirty-seven percent of the time, it is considered to be totally non-effective. Inert ingredients such as sugar pills or water injections often work because of the placebo effect. In other words, if one believes that something is going to work, it may well work for that individual.

The opposite is also true. Everyone in the medical profession knows that doctors, nurses, and their families are the worst patients. Not only are these people demanding, but they also know all the possible complications of their condition. Knowing what can go wrong makes it more likely to happen. Researchers have proven that if patients are given a list of all the possible side effects of their medications, they are more likely to experience those side effects. I guess this is one area where ignorance is helpful.

One of the first experiences I remember with the placebo effect was very dramatic. As a senior medical student, I served a preceptorship with a very knowledgeable physician in rural Kansas. One night we made a house call on a man named Frank who lived by himself. There had been a death in his family and Frank had not slept for several nights and had become very agitated. His family had called and asked us to help. On the way over we discussed the fact that Frank's problem was almost certainly emotional, as his family doctor knew him very well.

When we arrived, Frank recognized my preceptor, and I could tell that he had respect for him and believed in him.

After visiting for a few minutes, my preceptor said, "Frank, I'm going to have my assistant here give you a shot." Then, turning to me he said, "Dr. Old, give Frank here a shot."

"Sure," I replied, eager to do any type of medical procedure at that early stage of my medical training. "What do you want me to give him?"

"Oh," he replied, opening up his black bag and waving his hand across all the various vials of medication inside, "Just give him something out of here."

I wasn't sure what to do! I certainly didn't want to give him anything harmful. Finally I found a vial marked "sterile water." Even a medical student knows that couldn't harm anyone. So I carefully drew up two cc's of sterile water.

My preceptor leaned over to see what I had chosen. "Oh that is perfect!" he said reassuringly, with a slight wink.

Then looking Frank straight in the eye he told him, "Frank, it's eight o'clock now. As soon as we leave I want you to get ready for bed, because this is a strong shot. It's going to hit you in thirty minutes, and you will be out for the night. But make an appointment in the office tomorrow so I can check on you."

I gave Frank the shot, and we were on our way to make another couple of calls. I pretty much forgot about Frank until the next afternoon in the office when I saw him again with my supervising physician. As we entered the room Frank looked a little haggard, but well rested and not nearly as anxious. Before we could even ask anything, he jumped to his feet and proclaimed, "Doc, I really did something stupid last night."

"What was that?" asked my preceptor.

"Well," Frank continued, "I was feeling so up tight last night that I really didn't think that shot was going to do me much good, so I didn't get ready for bed like you told me to. I went into the kitchen to get something and noticed the stove clock. It said 8:30, and I suddenly remembered what you had said about the shot startin' to work then. All of a sudden it did kick in, and I got so sleepy I couldn't even walk out of the kitchen! I just collapsed right smack-dab in the middle of the kitchen floor, and slept there all night! Except for a stiff neck, I feel really good this mornin.' " Then, turning to me he said, "That sure was a powerful shot you gave me!"

I have never forgotten the power of the placebo effect! I use it often. Why not? I feel grateful for the ability of the human mind to fulfill expectations and to act on suggestions. Isn't the result what we are really interested in?

Vintage People seem to have mastered a way of positive thinking by using the placebo effect upon themselves. They believe in whatever they do for their health. If they take vitamin C every day to prevent colds—it probably does! If they walk every day for their health, it helps both physically and mentally. Beyond all else, I've found that Vintage People believe that they are blessed with good health. Even those with severe afflictions, when interviewed, feel that they are blessed with good health. They see the future for their health as bright. None of them bemoan the things they can no longer do because of health problems. They just ignore their chronic medical problems and truly believe in their own minds that their health is good. And it is!

Nutrition

We are what we eat! Vintage People realize the importance of nutrition in their health. "Eating right," "watching what I eat," and "eating fruits and vegetables," were listed as the top three factors when I asked Vintage People to explain their longevity. Many had developed creative ways of ensuring good nutrition.

Malnutrition becomes more common with aging for a number of reasons. As we age, senses of smell and taste often diminish, just as the sense of vision and hearing do. Foods don't taste as good. Medications often play a part in this as common prescription medications can give everything a "metallic" taste. Some medications, including common antacids, can impair the absorption of nutrients. Many social factors can also change the way we eat as we age.

"It's hard to cook good meals for just one person," writes one eighty-two-year-old Vintage Person. "After my husband died I had to force myself to continue cooking nutritious meals."

Shopping can be a problem. Transportation can become difficult, and neighborhood grocery stores that deliver are becoming a thing of the past. Many Vintage People are single. Even after they arrive at the large modern supermarket, it is hard to buy groceries for just one person. Supermarkets seldom package meats, bread, fresh vegetables, and other perishable products for single people. I learned this the hard way after becoming a single adult following a divorce. Hamburger comes in a one-and-one-half to a two-pound package. Fresh rolls and eggs are packaged by the dozen. Other foods also seem to be packaged for families—or for larger sales! About once a week I had to throw away a half package of green hamburger buns, a half loaf of moldy bread, and leftover fresh meats that had spoiled. (Yes, I know about freezing; I just prefer fresh foods!)

One Vintage Patient made an interesting observation. He told me that the advent of the salad and soup bar at the local foodliner had been a "godsend" for him. Finally he could buy just the right amounts of fresh fruits and vegetables that he could eat in one or two days before they deteriorated. At his suggestion, I, too, became a regular there at the deli bar during my single days.

Resourcefulness is common in Vintage People. Other tips these people follow include having nutritional snacks available and not skipping meals. Many of my patients who live alone cook regular size recipes, and then freeze or refrigerate several single-size portions to re-heat later. A Vintage Person I know often shares food back and forth with her neighbor, and they take turns cooking.

Adding spices and flavoring to foods is an important way to overcome the decreased acuity of the taste buds, which occurs with aging. After learning that ulcers and related diseases are not caused by these foods, physicians no longer prescribe the bland diets we once did for Vintage People. Many people need to limit salt in their diets, but many other seasonings are well tolerated and are not harmful to health. I like the "common sense" approach. I tell my patients that if a certain food bothers them, don't eat it. If it doesn't, then enjoy.

One of the best ways to insure good nutrition in the Vintage Person is to go to lunch or supper with a friend, a church group, or club. Pleasant social surroundings enhance the food. No medicines have been found that can stimulate the appetite like companionship can.

Chronic diseases

Not all Vintage People enjoy good health all the time. It would be naive to think that we are all going to be perfectly healthy as we age. However, I have found that Vintage People don't let physical problems interfere with their ability to enjoy life. I have mentioned my patient Jack before. He is paralyzed from the neck down. Yet he is an inspiration to many people in our town. He has a telephone headset and a way to dial by moving his chin. The ceiling of his bedroom is plastered with names and phone numbers which he can see from his bed without moving. Jack has undertaken the job of calling everyone in our church—about 500 members—on their birthdays. He also does other calling for the church such as reminding people of meetings. He helps with the "prayer chain" calling, often calling and praying with various people over the phone. He touches more lives from his bed and wheelchair than many of us who are ambulatory and in good health ever will.

Jack is just one of many Vintage People who are living their lives successfully in spite of a chronic disease or disability. Somehow they seem to ignore their defects. A homebound Vintage Person who reaches out from her home told me, "If I dwell on feeling bad, I feel bad. So I've just decided to be happy! I go on with my life, and as I do, I've found that my inability to walk really doesn't keep me from doing the things I want to do." She thought a few minutes and then added, "I guess I just have to want to do the right things!"

I promise to not get too medical here and will not describe all the various afflictions that affect mankind. Harrison's textbook of medicine has over two thousand pages, and it doesn't describe all of them.

We do not have cures for most chronic diseases. If our goal of curing all human disease can be compared to traveling to Mars, medical science has progressed to about the second story of a building. However there is one disease I want to mention because I find it to be fairly common and misunderstood. It is now easily treatable.

I'm referring to medical depression. The name itself is somewhat misleading. I am not talking about sadness or grieving. This is not the "blues." It is not the feeling I get when a lawyer wants to look at my medical records, or the feeling you got in high school when you saw your girlfriend with the captain of the football team or your boyfriend with the head cheerleader. Medical depression pushes you down. It is a feeling of hopelessness, a feeling of withdrawal. All pleasure in life is gone. A person with medical depression no longer looks forward to any of the things that he used to enjoy. Sleep is usually affected and patients feel worthless—even though there is no reason to have such a feeling. They are unable to concentrate and make decisions. With depression comes a severe chronic fatigue that won't go away. Thoughts of suicide and death often come up as part of this disease. The frustrating part is that everything in that person's life may be going well.

Often patients tell me they think they are going crazy. They also may feel that they are having a case of "wimphood!" They feel that they should be able to cheer themselves up or think their way out of the depression. After all, John Wayne could have lost the ranch, his girlfriend, and his best horse, and not suffered from depression. But you cannot think your way out of medical depression any more than you can think your way out of pneumonia. Not understanding the condition blocks treatment. And this disease can be fatal—suicide is a leading killer in all age groups.

We have recently discovered what causes depression. It is a chemical disorder just like low thyroid or diabetes. You cannot think or motivate your way out of physical disorders any more than you can depression. If we measure certain chemicals in the brains of depressed patients we find they are all deficient in the same chemicals. Fortunately, we have discovered how to put those chemicals back into the brain. When this is done, medical depression is controlled. Years of psychotherapy are not usually needed and a psychiatrist is not needed to treat this disorder. It now falls into the realm of the family doctor, who can treat it just like he would treat pneumonia or gout.

Depression affects our attitudes and the way we think. It can destroy the Vintage life-style quicker than most other physical afflictions. I want to stress that it is a disease, not part of normal aging! Older people do not naturally become depressed as they age. Depression is something to watch for and to treat. I have found that patients who have had medical depression before and know that it is treatable, will be back to see me when it begins to flare up. The disease is so miserable that they will seek treatment immediately.

Whether it is medical depression or other diseases, the good news is that the human body always tries to get back to its normal state. It has remarkable natural healing powers. Any physician can tell story after story of people who have recovered against all odds. Families often ask me "how long" a loved one has to live. I never put a time on something that variable. I have seen patients up eating and walking in the halls a few days after I thought there was no hope of survival. The Bible says we are "...wonderfully and mysteriously made." I have experienced that fact many times in my career. Vintage People always persevere in spite of chronic diseases.

Geriatric medicine

At eighty-seven years of age, George Burns wrote a national best-selling book entitled *How to Live to be One Hundred— or More.* In it he states: "Personally, I like an older doctor. And if he's still alive, I ask who his doctor is and go to him...if he's still alive. As soon as I find a doctor my age I'm going to keep him."

This statement points out a problem that has existed in the medical field. Older people present a different challenge that the medical profession is just now struggling to meet. Vintage People, as well as other older people, are not generic when it comes to health care. Our bodies change as we age, and we become a diverse group. Physicians must recognize that fact. Aside from our physical being, social situations and economic factors also change. A few numbers may help us understand the emergence of Geriatric Medicine. A child born in 1900 could expect to live an average of forty-seven and three-tenths years. A baby born in 1983 had a life expectancy of seventy-four and three-tenths years. By the year 2020 some predict life expectancy to be over eighty-five years. During the first part of this century, the increase in life expectancy was due largely to a decrease in the death rate of infants and children. Since about 1970, the increase has been due to decreased mortality in the older population.

People eighty-five and older constitute the fastest growing segment of our population. Some experts estimate that by the year 2050, fifty percent of the American population will live to celebrate their eighty-fifth birthday. In that year, the over eighty-five population will number approximately fifteen million.

The point is that we are an aging population, not just in this country but also world wide. In the United States now, twelve percent of the population is over the age of sixty-five. But they occupy eighty-eight percent of all nursing home beds, use forty-two percent of acute hospital days, and take thirty percent of all prescribed medications. Traditional medicine is having trouble keeping up with these changes.

As the numbers of older individuals increase, other factors get involved. Financial factors constitute one of the big concerns right now. The increasing older population is putting a huge demand on Medicare Trust Fund Reserves. Early in the 2000s, we may be dealing with negative numbers for Medicare funding. The deficit will become enormous as the demand for health care continues to increase. Let's look at the practical medical needs we are facing. Three factors affect our health as we age. First, there is biological aging—which is natural. This includes menopause, decreases in muscle mass, decreased strength, decreased physical reserves, and changes in gait. On top of these changes are those induced by disease. Examples are the effects of diabetes, arthritis, high blood pressure, cataracts, hearing loss, and a whole host of others. The third factor that affects aging is life-style. Abuses to our bodies over the years such as smoking—which definitely hastens aging—improper diet, alcohol, lack of exercise, obesity, inadequate sleep, and a number of other sins accelerate the aging process.

Social factors are also involved in the health-care of the older population. For starters, women outnumber men by far. Just at a time in life when companionship is needed, seventy-five percent of women find themselves alone. Society still seems to encourage women to marry older men, probably a holdover from the days when older men were better able to provide. In truth, women should probably be looking for a younger man who can care for them when they get older! On the flip side, psychologists tell me that women adapt to living alone much better that men do. Perhaps it all works out.

Because women live longer than men, on average, many Vintage People end up single. Most of these older single women live alone in their own homes or apartments. Ninety-five percent of us will never live in a nursing home, but a trade-off of not being in an institution is less access to health care. People who are institutionalized live in a central location with assigned caregivers. Living on their own, older single people face problems with availability of health care and transportation.

The hospital was once the center of the health care system. People were institutionalized and received care. I don't think that was a good system, but it was efficient. As a physician, I could make a few phone calls in the hospital and order physical therapy, rehabilitation, dentistry, podiatry, psychiatry and other disciplines to provide care for my patient. With the growth of managed health care in this country, the hospital is no longer in the center of health care. For a patient at home with the same condition formerly treated in the hospital, those services are harder to come by.

Removing the hospital as the primary source of health care is probably good. Most people are better off in their own homes and in familiar surroundings. Hospitals can be dangerous places for older people with decreased reserves. I've seen older patients undergo a vigorous prep for a barium enema, and then be required not to eat or drink for twelve to fifteen hours while awaiting results from their diagnostic tests. Delays are common. One older man I know became dehydrated while waiting for his X-rays to be completed. When he stood up, he became light-headed and fell, breaking his hip.

Anther problem with hospitals is that they are often noisy, and patients sleep poorly. Then there are all the medications—an average of seven to thirteen—that the hospitalized patient gets. Confusion is common, and accidents occur. Hospitals are also a great place to catch all kinds of germs. I don't want to scare anyone away from a hospital because it is great when needed, but stay away if you can, especially if you are older.

Home health agencies have sprung up all over. There are so many now that they compete for the same patients on a daily basis. The concept of home health care is great, the care is good, and it is less expensive than hospitalization. I am treating many illnesses at home now that would have been treated in the hospital fifteen years ago. However, it is not certain that there will be enough Medicare money to continue fully funding these operations as our population ages. Significant cutbacks have already started in determining which patients qualify for home health services under Medicare.

Physicians are learning more about the care of the elderly. The American Academy of Family Physicians sponsors excellent seminars on geriatric medicine. Geriatrics is now a required subject for all future family physicians during their residency training. There is even a board exam in geriatrics for physicians who wish to devote more of their energy to this field. All of this is paying off. We understand much more about the problems of aging than we did in the past.

In geriatric medicine we like to refer to "active life span" rather than total years of life. The major thrust in the practice of geriatrics today is to push disability toward the end of life as far as we can. For example, even though we cannot cure Alzheimer's disease, if we can delay its symptoms for five to ten years, many of the patients that it strikes will die from some other cause before they develop the disease and have that much more quality time. No one is going to live forever. Eventually we are all going to succumb to something, but a good quality of life in the years we live is a major objective in caring for Vintage People.

Physicians in geriatric medicine are working with their patients to add quality years to their life span. We are trying to put as much distance between birth and serious disability as possible. For example, we try to make sure that a person's home is as fall proof as possible. The home needs to be well lighted. Nutritious food needs to be available. Dentures may be imperative to nutrition and good health. Heat and cooling in the home is important as is cleanliness. Decreased hearing in the older individual is often misinterpreted by those around them as dementia, when in truth the person may just not be able to hear the question and respond appropriately. Hearing aids can help reduce this problem.

Life-style modifications are harder to achieve when we're older. Teaching and self discipline are essential. In this area true Vintage People stand out from "old people." Vintage People follow common sense practices such as a healthful diet, moderate exercise, and not smoking. They are aware of how their choices from day to day affect their health.

A third area in extending quality years to a person's life is the battle against disease. Prevention is best; treatment is next best. Many diseases such as diabetes can be deadly if not treated appropriately. The diabetic patient who learns to regulate his or her blood sugar can often eliminate complications of this disease or at least push them back further. Physical reserves diminish with age. The consequences of a bladder infection in a healthy twenty-year-old is generally minimal; the same infection in someone in their nineties may be fatal. Timely treatment of infections and diseases such as pneumonia are important.

Geriatric medicine requires a team approach to provide good care. I'm biased, of course, but I feel that family physicians are in the best position to direct that team. A number of parameters need to be covered. The home health agency, social services, medical equipment suppliers, dentists, podiatrists, nutritionists, mental health workers and even lawyers for estate planning, are needed to provide comprehensive care. The family physician and the patient's health care team can take care of eighty percent of the health problems that arise. Of course, physician specialists are needed to deal with specific medical problems such as cataracts, urinary problems, hearing loss, heart disease and other problems. Hospitals and nursing homes still play an important role, although the role of these institutions have been decreasing in recent years.

Geriatric medicine is becoming a specialty just like pediatrics or obstetrics. We are learning that Vintage People have unique needs and medical problems. Our approach to this set of patients is unique.

NINE

SEXUALITY AND INTIMACY

"Therefore a man leaves his father and his mother
and cleaves to his wife, and they become one
flesh."

—Genesis 2:24

One of my partners recently shared an amusing story
with me. He was called late one evening by a nurse at a
nursing home. She was so upset that she could hardly talk.
She had caught one of the older gentlemen in bed with one
of the female residents! She had no idea what to do!

"Well," inquired my partner, "Is either one of them
being hurt, or being forced to do anything against their
will?"

"Oh no," she replied, "They both seem to be really
enjoying each other!"

My partner's advice: "Shut the door and leave them
alone!"

The incident came up in the next regularly scheduled
meeting of nursing home directors. My partner and I were
trying to help the nursing home personnel keep such behavior in perspective and to propose ways to deal with such
incidents in the future. It was an emotionally charged area.
We thought we were making some progress until one of the
young administrators made a horrible face and said, "That's
really disgusting, don't you think?"

My partner's reply: "I don't think so! It kind of gives me hope!"

It should! Is it logical that healthy, vibrant people should suddenly give up their sexuality just because of advancing years? Blessed as I am with the medical care of a number of Vintage People, I have learned a lot about the importance of intimacy in their lives. As their doctor and their friend, I have been entrusted with many of their intimate secrets. I've learned that it is a myth that older people are not interested in sexuality. We are sexual beings and remain so throughout our lives.

The idea that sexuality stops at a certain age has been so widely propagated that even some of the senior citizens have started to believe it themselves—as if a decline in sexual activity is the norm. Look at the pictures of older people in magazines published several decades ago. (You can always find these magazines in your doctor's waiting room!)

At that time, Vintage People were portrayed as the grandmothers or grandfathers. Older men were stooped over with a cane. Older women looked like a painting of "Whistler's Mother," which is certainly not a sexual image. Today many of the ads in popular magazines and on TV show grandmothers in bathing suits; complete with makeup, jewelry and stylish hair, well tanned and playing with their grandchildren at the beach. Older men are often shown in a jogging suit, walking or riding a bike. This is quite a different picture from the old rocking-chair image!

It is a medical fact that 75 percent of males and 39 percent of women between the ages of 61 and 72 are sexually active. Partner availability obviously affects those statistics. The Starr-Weinder Report, published in 1981, revealed that when people from the ages of sixty to ninety-one were asked the question, "Would you like to have sex if it were available?" ninety-nine percent replied, "Yes!"

Other studies such as the Bretschneider-McCoy Study, in 1988 have shown sexual activity preserved in both men and women, to the age of 102! The loss of sexuality and intimacy is not a part of normal aging. Vintage People should not be expected to abandon their sexuality with advancing years. However, with maturity, the "rules" of sexuality change. And to my delight, and, I trust, to the delight of everyone reading this, Vintage People are telling me that it gets better!

Transformation

It is a biological fact that aging does cause some physical and psychological changes as far as sexuality is concerned. These are the normal changes of aging. Recent books— which have been very popular among Vintage People— detail these changes. Some of the most widely read include *Love and Sex After 60,* by Robert N. Butler, 1996; and *Questions and Answers About Sex in Later Life,* Margot Tallmer, editor, 1995. The most common normal physical change in women is vaginal dryness, a condition that is secondary to menopause and the loss of estrogen. This condition can be easily remedied by a water-soluble lubricant sold over the counter or by replacement hormone therapy.

For men, erections may not be as firm or as frequent with age, but they still occur. It is a misconception that a full, firm erection is needed for satisfying sex. If erections do not occur at all, it is not normal but the result of disease or medication. These conditions can usually be treated successfully. Several popular medications have just hit the market, and they work well.

I'm not going to detail all the physical changes that take place in this book. I highly recommend that you learn as much about your bodies as possible and believe that books on the subject are the best way to accomplish that. This is part of "Knowing Thyself." In this book I just want to stress that these are normal changes or transformations of aging and do not by themselves decrease a person's enjoyment of their sexual experience. Specific performance may be slower or altered, but total enjoyment may be enhanced. Vintage People have discovered this.

Situations that do interfere with sexuality include disease processes and life-style abuses—not part of normal aging. The medical profession is beginning to recognize this reality. I was at a medical seminar recently near a retirement community where a lot of Vintage People live. I was surprised by all the ads in the newspaper there concerning "impotence," "erectile dysfunction" (the politically correct term), and "sexual problems"! Without tremendous interest in these problems from this community of Vintage People, I doubt the urologists would spend that much on advertising. Viagra, by the way, outsold all other new prescription medications in history the first year it was introduced.

The good news is that even conditions caused by disease that interfere with sexual fulfillment usually can be helped medically. Many are simple to fix, as the urologists know. An informal "raise your hand" survey was conducted at a recent medical conference that I attended. The response indicated that almost one hundred percent of the physicians there are now using the "Viagra" test (giving the patient Viagra first, and if it doesn't work, then do the medical tests and work-up). Some are even using Viagra for women.

As they mature, Vintage People learn a lot about sexuality just as they discover new information in other areas of their lives. Whether in business, flying an airplane, raising children, fishing, doing household chores, golfing, or making love to your spouse, experience helps!

I am fortunate that my Vintage People have shared their valuable experience with me as their physician. A colleague attended a workshop a few years ago on "Sexual Medicine," during the Masters and Johnson era. "I came back so fired up," he told me. "I had been converted! I now realized how important it was to take a very detailed sexual history on all my patients! However, the first elderly lady that I asked explicitly about her sex life slapped me! And the second one replied, 'It's none of your business, Sonny!'"

I'm not sure how he approached the subject, and I realize he is in a different part of the country than I am, but my patients seem willing to talk honestly to me. One couple, the husband in his nineties and his wife eighty-seven, told me: "Sex has always been important to us. We have always been faithful to one another—even during the war while we were apart. We do things differently now than when we were young—there is a lot more hugging—but we enjoy it more now than ever."

This leads to a valuable point that I have learned from my Vintage Patients. In writing this chapter I have been careful to use the word "sexuality" and not just "sex." My Vintage Patients have taught me the immense difference in meaning between these two terms. They see a lot more to sexuality than just sex, or sexual intercourse. At this point the medical investigations and scientific data about sexuality begin to break down. All the scientific studies I have been able to find analyze such characteristics as the "number of times of intercourse per week," or the "number of erections in men," or the "frequency of orgasm" in women.

My Vintage Couples tell me that this type of information is missing the boat entirely. Genital sex is only one segment of overall sexual satisfaction! As they become Vintage

People, they realize that genital sex is a shrinking part of overall satisfaction. They have learned the broad, romantic definition of sexuality.

"Sexuality to me," wrote one Vintage Lady, "...involves so much more. So many young people overlook intimacy, love, closeness, bonding—just being with your best friend. To me sexuality also involves a morning cup of coffee together, a hug, watching a sunset, sharing a meal, sitting in church together; companionship...and sometimes just touching, and knowing someone loves you! There is so much more to it than just 'jumping into bed.' I'm not putting down the jumping into bed part, but my husband and I have learned that there is so much more as we have matured together."

What a beautiful view of sexuality! Vintage People have discovered something almost spiritual in sexuality. It involves intimacy. It touches the very human soul and involves the deepest sharing we will ever do with another human being. No wonder Donald Goergen wrote that "Sexuality and spirituality are not enemies but friends." This concept should give the rest of us something to look forward to.

Opportunities

"The retirement years are the best years for sexuality," writes a Vintage retired school teacher. "My husband and I are closer than ever. The kids have all moved out and the dog died! We have the whole house to ourselves and even though we both work part time, we have more time for each other."

Sexuality, intimacy, and closeness are a few of the pleasures of life, just like eating, smelling a rose, or looking at fine art. Vintage people see sexuality as something to be enjoyed to the fullest, and they have reached a time in life when they are free to partake of these pleasures. The kids are out of the house, and they are free to play and romance each other more. The pressures of work, school, children and financial worries are reduced. Often foreplay is longer and more romantic.

In Vintage People, sexuality involves more hugs, more cuddling and more touching than in many younger people, who want to race ahead for orgasm. But the kind of sexuality that Vintage People have discovered actually makes it better.

Vintage People are often creative in this respect. Most vintage couples that I interviewed had a "date night." That's something the new marriage manuals are just now recommending. These Vintage People figured it out on their own a long time ago. Many go out to eat, but others fix a special meal at home. Some go to a play, a movie, or just for a short walk. One wife, whose husband was in a wheelchair, wrote out a menu for him on Saturday nights, then served him a gourmet meal at home complete with candles and champagne. "It is important to do whatever it is that helped you fall in love in the first place," she explained. "Except now we can better afford it, we don't have to have our parents' approval, and we don't have to worry about getting pregnant!"

Other Vintage People just enjoy each other's company. They enjoy the love, the warmth, the closeness, and the feeling of knowing someone in the most intimate way. I think it is no accident that the Hebrew word for sexual intercourse is *yada,* which means "to know." The Old Testament often uses this term. The sexual experience involves vulnerability, sharing, and closeness. It somehow leads us into the mysterious sense of knowing each other as only lovers can.

The magic of the male-female relationship is indeed mystical, but we don't have to understand it to enjoy it! Romance is fully alive and well in the lives of Vintage People. An eighty-one-year-old Vintage Lady got right to the basis of what sexuality is all about when she said, "Above all, I think sexuality should be fun!" There it is, the bottom line about sexuality and intimacy. It is more than just procreation. It is more than a financial arrangement between husband and wife. It is more that dividing up household chores. Sexuality at its richest is fun; it is play; it is recreation. Couples get to know each other in a whole new playful way when the seriousness of the world is forgotten for a little while. They can delight in each other's companionship, and it can become a playful adventure. A Vintage Lady offered me this advice: "Tell your young married couples to stop reading those 'how-to' sex books. Most of them are so worried about doing everything right that they forget to just have fun!" Stated another way, C. S. Lewis said, "Banish play and laughter from the bed of love and you may let in a false goddess."

Obstacles

As we have seen, many Vintage People continue to enjoy sexuality and have actually learned to enhance it. Normal aging does not decrease this, and many of the diseases that affect sexuality are treatable. But there is one huge obstacle. Many Vintage People are without partners. Statistics show that women have a seventy-five percent chance of being a widow before they die. Being without a partner occurs less often for men, but is still common enough to present a problem. The biggest obstacle to sexuality and intimacy in the Vintage Person is often not a physical inability to perform. Disease does sometimes rob certain functions, but most couples can work around those. The biggest factor against enjoying sexuality and intimacy as a Vintage Person is lack of an appropriate partner.

A speaker at a medical seminar compared sexuality in the Vintage Person to riding a bicycle. There are several obstacles to overcome in both experiences as we age. First of all, there are increased physical limitations in both activities as we age. The muscles may get a little sore, and it may be a little more physically difficult to do either one. In addition to physical problems, there are social setbacks. Society judges Vintage People as looking silly on a bicycle, just as society does not expect sexuality in older people. By far the biggest obstacle to overcome is when someone takes away your bicycle! And that is what happens to a lot of Vintage People.

I'm amazed at how Vintage People deal with the loss of their "bicycle," as far as intimacy and sexuality is concerned. Some remarry. This is more common for men. Many choose to date but not to remarry. An eighty-two-year-old patient of mine writes, "I am so lucky to have known several wonderful gentlemen after I was widowed. Just having someone to travel with, to hold, and to share with has been wonderful!" The same lady explained to me that she would probably never remarry since she would lose her pension and because of other legal ramifications of inheritance.

Others remain celibate, either by choice or just because they don't meet the right person. Those who chose not to date also seem to be happy. I had a problem understanding this until one Vintage Man explained it to me like this. "I was married to Dottie for over fifty-four years. We shared children together, a lot of hardships together, and a lot of joys together. I know the love I felt for her can never be duplicated—I don't have enough years left to develop that kind of relationship. I don't feel guilty or feel like I would be betraying Dottie if I did date other women, but I just don't have any desire to. I like women as friends, but that's really all I'm interested in." Being happily married to a wonderful woman myself, I can relate to this feeling. It takes time to develop successful, intimate, sexually satisfying relationships, just like it takes time to develop Vintage People.

In spite of the obstacles, most Vintage People have used their creativity and powers of adapting to their present situation to arrive at a solution which meets their needs for sexuality and intimacy. And they have done it in spite of a sex-oriented society, that has ignored the sexual needs of its Vintage People.

God's sense of humor

Sexuality is uniquely human. Other animals experience reproductive sex, but not sexuality. When the female animal is not in heat, it is essentially non-sexual. Human sexuality combines reproduction, physical pleasure, love, and—I believe— even spirituality. What else has such a noble purpose?

Still, we don't have a clue as to what this "thing" we call sexuality is. Think how hard it would be to explain sexuality to someone from another planet where it did not exist. You would have to say something like this:

"There is this mysterious power that begins to influence human behavior early in life. There is no way to measure it, but it results in strange human rituals. Humans will make entirely irrational decisions because of it and give up great wealth in pursuit of it. Humans have been known to fight over it, and even kill because of it.

On the other hand, it can bring enormous joy and satisfaction. The existence of the entire Human species is dependent upon this "thing" which we can't even define. It makes rational men and women seek each other out, following some sort of mental and emotional check list that even they don't understand. Once they each find the "right" person, according to a vague checklist, which changes dependent upon the blood alcohol level, they may do some weird physical things to exchange some bodily fluids. Following this, two cells may combine into one cell inside the woman's body. This single new cell then changes into all the human parts, following a molecular blueprint that has been passed down since mankind began.

The new potential human starts out looking like a fish and is supported in fluid, the composition of which is similar to urine. It is linked to the outside world only by a tiny lifeline through which it receives all its life-sustaining nutrients. The new little human continues to grow inside the woman's abdomen, causing the organ that contains it to go from about the size of a pear to the size of an average bed pillow.

Finally, for yet unknown reasons, 280 days after it starts, this little human is propelled out of its dark, warm, fluid-filled environment. It enters the world about the size of a football, through a special passageway in the woman's body that is only just big enough for a ping-pong ball to pass. But despite all the squeezing and contorting it does to get out, it seems to do very well.

At the instant that the little human comes into the world, its entire circulatory and respiratory systems have to change as it transforms from an aqueous organism to a land-dwelling, air-breathing baby. When born, it is totally helpless and totally inconti- nent. It can't feed itself, adequately warm itself, or move about in its environment. It is completely dependent upon other humans for its survival requir- ing around-the-clock care. In appreciation for all the care, it returns essentially nothing to the humans who care for it except for dirty diapers and lots of crying.

And upon all of this the very existence of the human species is dependent."

Our alien listening to this explanation would likely say; "Yeah! Right! Now tell me what really happens!"

To me, the whole area of sex, sexuality, and reproduc- tion proves that God does indeed have a sense of humor. Somehow our sexuality makes us what we are and links us to God in a spiritual sense. God created sexuality and then proclaimed that it was good. In some mysterious way, both males and females are created in "His own image." We are both created in the image of God and are therefore both drawn together spiritually.

TEN

HUMOR

"A merry heart doeth good like a medicine."
—Proverbs 17:22

This may be the most important chapter of this book. I have found humor to be such an important characteristic of Vintage People that I am willing to say that without it we cannot be successful in aging. At the very least, the power that comes from aging will be diminished if we don't develop a sense of humor. We can get old without a sense of humor, but we cannot be a Vintage Person without seeing the whimsical side of life.

All of us like to laugh. The reason is simple—it makes us feel better. As early as four months of age, babies begin to laugh. If we are lucky, laughter is one of the last gifts we lose at the other end of life. God seems to feel that laughter is one gift that is important to our well-being throughout our lives. A sense of humor is something all Vintage People agree is important to longevity and successful living.

The Vintage People I interviewed broke their sense of humor down into two important parts. First was the ability to laugh at the absurdities of life and to take things a little less seriously. The second segment was the ability to laugh at themselves. Vintage People have found that humor helps them to stay flexible and in control. It helps them adapt, to stay healthy mentally and physically, and to remain creative in the face of difficulty and disasters.

Vintage People believe that a sense of humor can be developed by anyone—it is a learned skill. We have control over our own sense of humor. It's not something we either have or don't have or an inherited, genetic characteristic as many people believe. Most of the Vintage People in my studies had not been gifted with a sense of humor. The majority had tough lives filled with pain and loss—hardly an arena for developing a sense of humor. But they learned to cope. They developed a way of looking at life that removed the seriousness and despondency. They developed a sense of joy in being alive, even when the world didn't want to cooperate. One Vintage Banker told me, "You might just as well learn to laugh at all the things that go wrong, because they are going to happen anyway!"

Vintage People have learned the secret of humor.

Laughter is good for your health

A physician by the name of Norman Cousins discovered the physical benefits of laughter while a patient himself, suffering from severe pain secondary to the inflammation of his spine and joints. It was painful for him to move. He discovered that laughter was good medicine. He found that ten minutes of solid laughter would give him about two hours of pain-free sleep. He began watching comedy tapes such as old Marx Brothers films and found the benefits of laughter greater than that of pain medications and narcotics. He named his discovery "laugh therapy" and published a book about it.

Subsequent studies have proven the pain-killing effects of laughter. It has been discovered that with laughter certain chemicals called endorphins are created in the central nervous system. These chemicals are the body's natural pain killers. When released into the body's circulation, endorphins have a pleasing effect on the mind and a numbing effect on pain. It is cheap medicine.

Laughter is also good physical exercise for the body. Some of the changes are obvious. When we laugh, our fifteen facial muscles change positions and alter our physical appearance. Heart rate and blood pressure increase so that circulation carries more oxygen and nutrients to all the tissues of the body. It is estimated that one hundred chuckles a day—the average for most joyful adults—is equivalent to riding a stationary bike for fifteen minutes or spending ten minutes on a rowing machine.

The initial effects of laughter are stimulating, followed by a period of relaxation and a sense of well being. The next time you experience a prolonged belly laugh, notice that afterwards you take a deep breath—and sigh—reflecting a release of tension. In short, it makes us feel better and more relaxed. Have you ever watched children when they are really laughing? They hold their sides and even roll to the floor with laughter. That is because all the muscles relax, and they are unable even to stand. This behavior is not becoming for adults, but you can probably remember doing that as a child, and that it made you feel good! Aristotle said that "laughter is a bodily exercise precious to health." *Reader's Digest,* one of the most popular and widely read magazines of all time, has a section called "Laughter, the Best Medicine." If I could bottle laughter, what a remarkable, all-purpose medicine I would have.

One of the first characteristics we lose at the beginning of any mental illness is our sense of humor and joy of living. This occurs at the onset of most physical illnesses as well. Ask any obstetrician or obstetrical nurse (or husband) about how women in labor seem to lose their sense of humor as labor progresses. Almost all pregnant women who are in early labor enter the hospital excited and jovial. That takes a nasty turn by the time they are dilated six or seven centimeters! I can personally relate to this. I recently had a kidney stone and quickly lost my sense of humor! Good health and joy are closely linked to humor.

If good health and feeling well can create humor and laughter, can the opposite also be true? Can laughter, and a sense of humor make you feel joyful, and even lead to good health? Research in the field of psychoneuroimmunology (the study of the mind, body, and immune systems), suggests that it can. This new field of study, which wasn't recognized until 1981, suggests that laughter can not only make us feel happier, but it can even affect our immune systems—our sensitivity to disease! People who use humor in their lives tend to have an enhanced immune system. In one study, people who were in high stress occupations were divided into two groups—those who used humor to help handle their stress and those that did not. It was found that those who use humor to cope had higher levels of immunoglobulins—infection fighting substances. In another study it was found that the levels of immunoglobulins increased after subjects watched a humor video, but did not increase in people who watched an instructional video.

I'm not suggesting that humor and laughing can cure pneumonia or appendicitis, but science is beginning to realize the benefits of humor in medical treatments. Merriment, just like regular physical exercise, good nutrition, and proper sleep, can help keep one's mind and body in optimum medical shape. It can help prevent illness, and if illness does occur, it can help with healing. I believe there is a lot of fun in medicine, but there is also a lot of medicine in fun. Vintage People have learned this fact.

Mental attitude

Not only can laughter make us feel better physically, it also affects us mentally and spiritually. It is impossible to be angry, depressed, or resentful, when we are laughing. Laughter relieves the strain of the day. Niels Bohr, the renowned nuclear physicist who discovered the basic atomic structure of nature says, "There are some things so serious that you have to laugh at them."

I experienced this first hand as I went through my medical training. I noticed that often during a medical crisis, one of the doctors or nurses would make a humorous remark. At first I was appalled. Someone's life is hanging in the balance here, and the noble medical professionals who are supposed to be caring for them are poking fun? But soon I realized that this is a coping mechanism commonly seen in stressful situations. In the medical profession the most common places for laughter are the emergency rooms and in surgery. Those are often the areas of highest stress as well.

A few years ago a young man was brought to the emergency room after being shot in the head during a poker game. (Yes, that still happens in Kansas!) Several of the staff, including myself, knew the young man and his family. It was extremely difficult for all of us, as there was nothing we could do to save him. A couple of hours later, we were in the staff room talking and laughing about something totally unrelated to the situation. The door was open and a patient who had been placed next door for a minor aliment walked into the staff room, furious. "Someone was just killed here and you are laughing!" he yelled.

I'm sure he never understood the reasons for our laughter in this situation, but it was a form of release, of therapy for the staff involved. No harm or callousness was intended. I have since found that laughter is used in almost all high-stress occupations. When I have been invited to visit police stations, fire stations, and even military installations—anywhere tensions run high—there is silliness and laughter during the idle times. It is a coping mechanism learned by these professionals. Mohandas Gandhi said, "If I had no sense of humor, I should long ago have committed suicide." So it is in situations of high stress and high human discipline.

Research shows that people who use humor in their lives, suffer less tension, anger, fatigue, and depression than others. Certainly in treating patients, physicians who can see the absurdity in difficult situations, such as illness and aging, seem to be happier and more successful at whatever they try. They are less likely to be bored with life and less likely to "burn out" in their professions. Physicians who are serious all the time are less satisfied with their jobs and their lives. Those who laugh; those who have fun with their patients and staff; those who can see the absurdity of Medicare bureaucrats, insurance companies, hospital administrators, and even illnesses themselves; all of these seem to be more successful at the practice of medicine and at life. They are more fun to be around and have better mental and physical health.

I've heard about a group of doctors at a nearby Catholic hospital who were known to be jesters. Occasionally obstetrical patients who were delivering by C-section would request to have a tubal ligation sterilization done at the same time instead of having another surgery later. Sterilization was not allowed in the Catholic hospital, but this group of physicians had figured out a way to beat the system. A nun would stand in the operating room during the surgeries to be sure sterilizations were not done. If the patient had requested the procedure from this group of doctors, nothing was said. But when they neared that part of the operation, one or the other of the surgeons would start to use all kinds of foul language. Offended, the nun would step out of the room, and they did the tubal ligation!

I think Vintage People have also discovered how to use humor as a coping mechanism without belittling anyone or anything. Humor seems to be especially helpful in counteracting the changes of aging. As one Vintage Lady told me, "I used to think that the 'humor of aging' was an oxymoron, but as I got older I now think it is a good description of the whole aging process." America uses humor to help us cope, collectively, as a nation. I'm amazed at how jokes pop up about some of our most serious and "unfunny" national stories. Look at the O.J. jokes! There are jokes about the Titanic, about President Clinton and his White House interns, and even about the Oklahoma City bombing. No one that I have ever heard repeat one of these jokes doubts the seriousness of the related situations. Nor do they mean any disrespect to those people involved. It is quite the opposite. They are so overwhelmed by the even thought of these losses that they need a mechanism to cope. And that is where humor comes in.

Bill Cosby once said, "You can turn painful situations around through laughter. If you can find humor in anything, you can survive it." Ironically, this quotation was written years before the tragic murder of his only son along an interstate highway in California. But Mr. Cosby was able to follow his own advice and provided a great lesson to the American people following his tragic loss. I'm paraphrasing here, but in an interview shortly after the unfortunate event, he said something like this: "I must go on. I'm a comedian and I must make people laugh, for laughter is important. Everyone has experienced some form of tragedy in their lives—some probably worse than mine—but it is important that we all go on laughing and living our lives. I'm just glad that God let me know Him!"

Most great leaders have recognized the value of laughter. Biographers tell us that Abraham Lincoln, even during the strain of the Civil War, took time to laugh. Richard Hanser, writing about Lincoln in 1952, says that, "Humor was his bulwark against the bitter and bloody disasters of the Civil War. His gaunt, towering figure, clad in flapping flannel nightgown, used to stalk through the White House at midnight seeking someone still awake to share a funny story he had just read."

It is reported that at one time during the bleak days of the Civil War, during the meeting of the War Cabinet, Mr. Lincoln started the meeting by reading a funny story. When he was finished, he laughed heartily. Members of the War Cabinet were furious! These were serious times! Didn't the president understand that? But Mr. Lincoln stood up, looked them straight in the eye, and said, "Gentlemen, why don't you laugh? With the fearful strain that is upon me night and day, if I did not laugh, I should die, and you need this medicine as much as I do." It was at this same meeting that he presented the Emancipation Proclamation—hardly a light document!

Humor also has much to do with creativity. The Latin root of the word, *umor,* actually refers to "fluid." Medical texts early in this century often referred to the aqueous humor, or fluids of the body. Even the word itself has to do with flexibility. A sense of humor helps distance us enough from a problem that we can see other alternatives. If our mind is focused on only one thing—the worst problem that has ever happened—it is hard to think of anything else. With humor the urgency and seriousness of the problem is dispelled. Is this the worst problem the world has ever seen? Probably not! We begin to realize the absurdity of the problem and of our reaction to it. At that point, the mind can become more open, more flexible, and more creative. I know that in tense medical situations, if I can make a humorous comment, the nurses and other medical staff often begin to relax, and everyone begins to think and function better. Humor can be a powerful tool for staying in control of a situation.

Humor relieves stress. If you have ever tried to talk to a room full of teenagers about responsible sex, you will hear a lot of nervous giggling and humorous comments. Using humor relieves the tension of the moment. This will work in business, at school, at church, or wherever stress levels soar. Vintage People realize that life is not a bowl of cherries. There are painful times. But these people have learned to react with a sense of humor that helps them cope and remain creative and flexible.

Human relationships

Using humor to foster human relationships is an area where Vintage People have excelled. They know that humor often helps diffuse otherwise potentially dangerous situations. Vintage People have become skilled at making a point, without having people take offense. One Vintage Gentleman that I saw a few days ago told me as I entered the exam room at 4:30 for his 3:15 appointment: "I'm sorry you didn't get to see me sooner Doc," he said, "but I got hung up in your waiting room!" I got the point, and neither of us had to be upset or angry.

Famous people have used these techniques as well. One time, when a heckler called President Lincoln two-faced, the president retorted, "If I'm two-faced, would I be wearing this one?"

When I first started my medical practice in a small Kansas town, I found that people stopped me at church, at the grocery store, and wherever else I might be, for medical advice. I asked one of the semi-retired physicians who still practiced part-time in our group how he handled that situation. After all, he had lived here for over forty years. "Well," he replied, "I learned how to handle that a long time ago. Whenever someone asks me a medical question outside the office, I just tell them that if they will take all their clothes off right there, I will examine them. If they prefer to wait, I will see them in the office. So far, I've not had anyone disrobe in church!" He used humor to get his message across, and did not offend the patient in the process. I've used that now for years, and it works!

Dr. Albert Schweitzer is reported to have told jokes and amusing stories to his staff during the dinner hour to nourish their spirits while working in deplorable conditions. Winston Churchill, John F. Kennedy, and Dr. Martin Luther King, Jr., all used a sense of humor in their leadership roles. Even Jesus had a sense of humor which is revealed in many of his parables. Charles Schultz says, "No one would have been invited to dinner as often as Jesus was unless he was interesting and had a sense of humor."

Research has shown that humor brings us together as humans. It increases bonding and camaraderie. Watch children playing. Watch teenagers at a party. You will observe all kinds of silliness, giggling, and laughter. But what are they really doing? They are communicating; they are sharing the uniquely human characteristic of humor. And they feel a glowing sense of belonging, a sense of being accepted, and a sense of joy in life. Friends are being made. Researchers have found that this process can spill over into the work place. Humor on the job has been shown to increase productivity, teamwork, and cooperativeness.

Humor is also great at diffusing difficult situations. Consider the story told by Malcolm Kushner in *The Light Touch: How to Use Humor for Business Success,* Simon &

Schuster, 1990. A police officer was investigating a routine domestic disturbance call—a husband and wife fight. As she parked her patrol car in front of the offenders' house, a television flew out of a second-story window. Loud voices argued as she walked to the front door and knocked. An angry man screamed, "Who is it?" The officer knew that if she said "Police," it would only make things worse. Instead, she replied "TV repairman!" The man started laughing and opened the door. The first step in resolving the dispute had been taken.

A surgeon I knew used humor to dispel his patients' anxiety before surgery. He would always discuss the procedure in detail with them days before, but on the morning of surgery he would visit them just prior to them going into the operating room. He would make comments such as, "Now what was I going to do to you? Was it castration?" This was usually followed by the patient laughing and explaining the procedure back to him, which helped to prove that the patient understood the intended procedure. Then he would say, "Gosh, I hope I can remember how to do that. Maybe I had better have the nurses get my book out!" Of course the patients totally trusted his skills, but his humor helped to relieve their tension. When these patients returned to me for follow-up care, the surgeon's humorous comments were usually the main things that they remembered about their surgery.

The people that make commercials have learned that next to sex humor sells. It is a universal language that every one seems to enjoy. Vintage People have learned that humor is a uniquely human trait that tends to bring people together. It encourages good human relationships. They use it as a tool in getting along with other people.

Vintage People laugh at themselves

Of all the benefits of laughter, probably the most powerful one that Vintage People have learned is the ability to laugh at themselves. Will Rogers says, "Everything is funny as long as it's happening to somebody else." But what about when it happens to us? This is where God has given us a great coping mechanism—the ability to laugh at ourselves. And other people love it when we can laugh at ourselves. This skill is invaluable in human relationships, but we must learn to use it. Edith Barrymore says, "You grow up the day you have your first real laugh at yourself."

I have a large cottonwood tree in front of my house that has grown bigger each year. Its roots were beginning to push up my sidewalk, and I was afraid that with a storm it would split and fall on my house. So I decided many months ago that it had to be cut down. There is a large space in the driveway where it could fall. I planned how to cut it down carefully and even waited until the wind was in the right direction. I put a rope on it and pulled it in the direction I wanted it to go with the tractor. I notched the tree and had everything prepared to fall to the north. However, it fell instead many feet to the south of my objective, dragging my tractor with it and crashing into the house! The very thing that I feared and hoped to prevent by cutting the tree had just happened!

My wife and daughter ran out in horror to see what the crash was. As I stood there with the chain saw in my hand, it was pretty hard to deny what I had done. After the initial shock and anger passed, I knew I had to make a decision. As I stood there wanting to cry and to cuss, I made a conscious decision to see it as funny. After all, everyone else from the insurance adjuster, to the carpenter, to the gutter repair person, would think it was funny. "Doc cut a tree and let it fall on his house," I could hear them say. "I hope you are a better people surgeon than tree surgeon!" "You better stick to doctoring!" "I always thought you were smarter than a tree!"

"Why should I let them have all the fun!" I thought to myself. I might as well laugh at myself, too. Once I made that decision, I found I was not nearly as upset. Standing there in disbelief I uttered, "I hate it when that happens!" Then I started laughing, as my wife and daughter joined in. Deciding to view it as funny changed the way I felt! The anger disappeared, and I was able to look at the situation more objectively. It no longer seemed like the end of the world. No one was hurt, and the house could be fixed. And besides, I had insurance! Laughing at myself let me in on the fun too. I have found that to be a tremendous coping mechanism.

We don't have to wait for a tree to fall on our house to see things as funny. If we look, we do funny things all the time. Maybe we have the best organized—or the junkiest—garage in the neighborhood. How about the way we use the "good dishes" only on special occasions. My wife and I have a standing joke about eating in the dining room. For some reason we usually eat in the kitchen. Whenever we eat in the dining room, we borrow a line from the TV commercial several years ago: "So, this is the dining room!"

My partner told me about a Vintage Patient he saw in the office recently. He had been treating her asthma with an inhaler for several months. He had given her several different inhalers, but to his surprise none seemed to work very well on her condition. Finally her daughter came with her for an office visit. After listening to her lungs he discovered that she was finally breathing much better. My partner remarked that a type of inhaler had been found that seemed to be helping her asthma. The older lady looked at her daughter and said, "Shall we tell him?"

"Oh no," replied the daughter. "Don't tell him."

"Come on," said my partner. "You can't leave me hanging like that. Tell me what?"

"Well, okay," she started, "I had been using those inhalers for several weeks and none of them seemed to be doing any good at all. One afternoon my daughter was visiting me, and I asked her to hand me the inhaler so I could take my dose of medicine. I started to take it out of her hand and she said, 'Wait mother, and I will take the cap off for you.' 'Cap,' I replied, 'What cap?!' It worked a lot better after I learned to take the cap off!"

Then mother and daughter both leaned back and laughed enthusiastically. Obviously this Vintage Lady was able to laugh at herself, and she was enjoying the funny story more than anyone! That characteristic seems to be paramount in successful Vintage People. Laughing at oneself is truly good medicine. As one eighty-six year-old Vintage Lady told me, "Doc, since I have learned to laugh at myself, I've never had to worry about being entertained!"

Learned humor

Humor seems to be a skill that can be learned. Many Vintage People tell me that they had to develop the ability to take themselves a little lighter, and to see life as humorous and joyful. Unfortunately, many people relate a "sense of humor" to someone who seems to have a God-given talent to pop off one wisecrack after another. That is only a very small part of a sense of humor. Laughing is another part. Many people can have a terrific sense of humor but not laugh much. By the term "sense of humor" I am talking about a perspective of life, a way of dealing with problems and hardship, a way of staying in control of situations, and a way of finding joy in life. This can be learned, developed and practiced.

Abraham Lincoln said, "I've noticed that most people are about as happy as they make up their minds to be." He realized that we do indeed have a choice. When bad things happen, we can choose to stand back and view life as a joke. It may not be something that we laugh out loud about, but if our overall perspective of life is one of gladness, joy, and delight, then we are approaching it with a sense of humor. Our thoughts, our perspectives, our attitudes make a tremendous difference in how we feel. Humor is a big part of our wellness system.

How do we choose to be happy—to enjoy a sense of humor? Sometimes we may not feel funny. At times we don't feel like looking for the funny side of anything. How do Vintage People develop this skill? The key is in the way the human mind works. William James of Harvard University, the father of American psychology, explained it this way, "The greatest discovery of my generation is that human beings can alter their lives by altering their attitudes of mind." This profound statement shows the tremendous potential we have to be happy. We don't have to see things the same way that someone else does. We don't even have to accept any event as negative. All of us have the power in our minds to turn almost anything around and view it as funny or positive. We have the power to "lighten up" and look for the joy of living.

Earlier I described the human mind as being somewhat like a computer. That is only part of the story. Our mind can store facts like a computer. But unlike any computer, our human minds also store feelings and emotions. The marvelous human mind draws upon all stored facts as well as feelings and emotions to create thoughts. Through a complicated process, thoughts become the basis of our actions. Simply stated, our actions are based on facts as well as perceived facts, emotions, and feelings. The reverse is also true. Our actions influence our feelings. In short, if we act happy, happiness will often follow. One of the Proverbs says, "When a man is gloomy, everything seems to go wrong; when he is cheerful, everything seems right!" (Living Bible translation.)

One day while seeing my patients at a local nursing home, I could hear Ruby moaning all the way down the hallway. I had known Ruby for some time and knew that she always saw everything in the worst possible way. She was a frail, gloomy, petite lady with arthritis that caused her considerable pain. When I finally approached her, she began moaning even louder. The nurse whispered to me, "That's just Ruby! She refuses to take any of her pain medications."

Finally I walked up to Ruby, and asked how she was. "Terrible," she exclaimed, and continued moaning.

"If you are so uncomfortable, why don't you take your pain medications?" I asked.

I will never forget her answer because it was so honest. "If I do that," she said, "no one can tell how much I am suffering!"

Attitudes can affect all of us. In medical school, there was a traditional "trick" played on a new medical student on the psychiatry service each semester. The first day he or she was there, the interns, residents, and other staff members would all comment one by one that he or she looked sick. The first one would ask, "Do you feel okay? You don't look too good." At first the student would reply that he or she felt fine. But as the day wore on, more and more people would comment that he looked ill. By the time evening rounds came, the student had invariably gone home sick! After he had "recovered," the experience was used as a teaching device to help us see how the human mind works. You can make yourself sick by your thoughts, and you can also make yourself well by your thoughts.

This great capacity of the human mind is how Vintage People have learned to see life in a humorous and joyful way. They purposefully put happy, pleasant thoughts in their minds. When negative thoughts interrupt, they have a favorite saying or vision to replace it. "Whenever something upsets me," writes one grandmother, "I just think of my grandchildren and the fun we had the last time we were together. Then whatever it was doesn't seem nearly as important." Another lady told me, "When I'm trying to go to sleep and my mind is full of all the bad things that may have happened during the day, I imagine myself at the beach, with the soothing sound of the waves breaking. Why, I can even feel the warmth of the sunshine!" These Vintage People have learned the power of thoughts. What we think about often determines our moods. Think happy, pleasant, cheerful thoughts, and you will feel that way. As Ralph Waldo Emerson said, "A man is what he thinks about all day long."

Vintage People realize that their actions have to do with the way they feel. And they realize they have control over their actions. For example, if you don't feel like smiling, smile anyway. In a little while you may feel like smiling or laughing. We use this principle with children all the time. "Smile!" you tell a crying child. Once they do, even though they don't want to, the hurt begins to fade and they are soon laughing. There is a saying that those who work in addictions use. Patients are taught to rehearse it in their minds. If they feel they are about to lose control and get into trouble, they are taught to "Fake it until you make it!" In other words, act as though you are strong, and you often will be

171

surprised at how strong you turn out to be. Act as though you are happy, and soon you may realize that you are.

Sharing humor with others is another proven method of adding joy to your life. Joking with family members, friends, coworkers, and even strangers, is uplifting. Silliness is good for you. The word silly comes from the Old English word *saelig* which means happy, prosperous and blessed. So silly is not stupid! In our society silliness is sometimes associated with lack of intelligence. But you don't have to be a raging "ding-bat" to enjoy life with a sense of humor. A lot of entertainers, speakers, writers, and advertising agents, have made a great deal of money from "silliness." Being silly does not mean you lack intelligence. We have eight Board Certified Family Physicians in our group, and you wouldn't believe some of the silly things that come over our fax every day. One of the most popular medical journals we receive contains numerous medical cartoons dispersed among the articles. Humor is contagious when it is shared.

The final characteristic that helps Vintage People develop a sense of humor is the fact that they don't worry much about what other people think. They have gotten past that. They have learned that there are people who will agree with whatever you do, and people that will disagree with whatever you do, so you might just as well do what you want to do. As George Burns said, "At my age there isn't much peer pressure!" Vintage People have reached a freedom to be silly, to laugh, and to enjoy life. One of the most touching stories about how Vintage People can enlighten their lives with humor came from the great playwright Oscar Wilde. He was able to use humor even as he lay dying, when he is reported to have quipped: "My wallpaper and I are fighting a duel to the death. One or the other of us has to go!"

ELEVEN

ENJOY THE MOMENT

"For yesterday is already a dream,
And tomorrow is only a vision;
But today, well-lived,
Makes every yesterday a dream of happiness
And every tomorrow a vision of hope.
Look well, therefore, to this day!"

—Anonymous

I love the story I heard a speaker tell about the optimist who was visiting the Empire State Building in New York. He was so enthralled by the view and the majesty of the building that he lost his balance and fell off the top. As he was falling, people were reaching out of windows trying to catch him. But they kept missing. As he sped past they could hear him say, "I'm Okay—so far!"

Now that man was an optimist! He was also enjoying the moment. He was living each second in the present. He wasn't worrying about the future. Almost every moment of our lives, we are okay. And it is amazing how many moments we can get through when we view it that way.

I have found that Vintage People have this outlook towards life. They tend to worry less about the past and less about the future than the rest of us. They know they are forgiven for mistakes in the past. They don't worry about what the neighbors think. And they don't dwell on all the things that could happen in the future. They tend to "take life an inch at a time," and just enjoy the moment. And by enjoying the moment, they put power in their future and make it brighter as well.

Forgiving the past

Vintage People have learned it is not in their best interest to carry a grudge. Stated another way, Vintage People seem to be very forgiving. They have learned a great principle of life. By carrying a grudge, living in guilt, or failing to forgive, the past is reaching out and ruining the present. They cannot enjoy the moment if haunted by the past. Vintage People have learned that this is a major roadblock to happiness and success. Jesus taught this fact of human interaction two thousand years ago. Today's psychologists are just now re-discovering it. We forgive another, not for their sake, but for our own sake. It may seem ironic, but forgiving someone makes the forgiver feel good, whether or not it helps the one who is forgiven. The enemy may not even know that he has been forgiven, but a great feeling of peace comes over the forgiver. There is an ancient Chinese proverb which states, "The best way to get even with your enemy is to forgive him!"

Similarly, when we can put to rest a grudge, resentment, or revenge, it no longer has any power over our future. Whenever any of this negative baggage affects the present, we are under its control. The past is not only reaching out and dragging us down in the present, but it is blocking our future as well.

Several years ago I attended a divorce workshop taught by a minister. I remember him asking the room full of emotionally hurting, recently divorced adults, "What is the opposite emotion from love?"

Immediately several people shouted out, "Hate!"

"No," he explained. "Both love and hate are powerful emotions that control our lives. The opposite of love is indifference—not caring."

What he was talking about is becoming neutral. As long as we have any strong emotional attachments, either love or hate, those emotions will control what we do in the present. The past is controlling what we do in the moment. In divorce, as in many other situations in life, until there is complete forgiveness—until we arrive at being indifferent—then the past still controls and significantly hampers our enjoyment of the present, and it is difficult to go on with our future.

Another common roadblock to enjoying the moment is guilt. Guilt is one of the major emotions that robs people of happiness. I see this almost daily in my practice. Guilt is often a major player in patients with stress; in patients with anxiety; in patients with depression; even in patients who contemplate or accomplish suicide. What is guilt? Put simply, it is a lack of forgiving ourselves. It is resentment, or carrying a grudge against ourselves. And many times self-forgiveness is one of the hardest forms of forgiveness.

One Vintage Lady explained a unique way of self forgiveness to me. "A long time ago," she stated, "I felt guilty about so many things. I knew that God would forgive me, and I prayed every day for that to happen. But I never felt forgiven. Then one day it just hit me. In the Bible God said He would forgive me if I asked, and I had asked. If I didn't believe I was forgiven, then it was Satan making me feel that way. Once I looked at it that way, I was able to forgive myself and go on with my life."

Lack of forgiveness can make us miserable. Forgiveness can make life wonderful. That is what led the apostle Paul to write, "Forgive as freely as the Lord has forgiven you" (Colossians 3:13). Forgiveness and the lack of forgiveness, can even affect our health—mental, spiritual, and physical.

A task I am sometimes called upon to perform is to review potential medical malpractice cases for certain insurance carriers. I'm amazed at how people handle bad situations differently. A potential case I reviewed a number of years ago involved a woman who had awakened from anesthesia during a surgical procedure. Since modern anesthesia involves totally relaxing all the muscles of the body, the woman could not move, talk, or signal anyone she was awake. Obviously this was a dreadful, frightful, and painful experience that no one should have to endure. The anesthesiologist was unaware of her condition because he did not have monitoring equipment to alert him to such a circumstance.

Everyone involved felt horrible about what had happened and feared the worst. The insurance company was surprised however, when this patient refused to sue anyone. Instead she began to crusade for hospitals to purchase and use monitors that would prevent this terrible event from happening to anyone else! She was determined to make something good come out of a bad situation. This woman recovered quickly from her surgery and focused her energy in a positive way. She felt good about herself and the message she had to give. She had forgiven the past, was living in the moment, and had hope to change the future.

This story stands in sharp contrast to experiences of people who focus on their pain, catastrophes, and bad outcomes. It is a known medical fact that patients who are involved in lawsuits, either with workers' compensation or medical malpractice, get well much more slowly than those who are not. Patients involved in litigation dwell upon their misfortunes, and these negative thoughts slow their healing. Even if their financial incentive to stay sick is removed, these patients have been shown to suffer more and to be more unhappy than those who can forgive and go on with their lives.

I am not trying to justify or excuse medical malpractice, but rather to make a point about dwelling on past torments. Vintage People have learned to control this. They don't let the past reach into their present. This principle caused E. H. Chapin to write, "Never does the human soul appear so strong and noble as when it forgoes revenge and dares to forgive an injury." One of my Vintage Patients stated it this way, "The greatest pleasure you can experience is the feeling that comes over you when you truly forgive an enemy—whether he knows it or not."

Forgiveness can be compared to a painful wound. When the wound is fresh, it festers and is painful. Resentment and revenge keeps the wound open and forces us to "re-feel" the pain. With forgiveness the wound is allowed to heal into a tough scar. Most scars are permanent and serve as a reminder to not forget completely, but with forgiveness the scars are no longer painful. We don't truly recover until we forgive.

Vintage People seem to have learned this lesson well. They are forgiving, whether they recognize it or not, for their own well-being. They have the ability to put all sorts of bad things behind them, forgive, and go on with their lives. Ann Landers sums up what I am talking about when she writes, "One of the secrets of a long and fruitful life is to forgive everybody, everything, every night, before you go to bed."

The unforgiving person is taking on a burden that even God chose not to embrace.

One day at a time

Vintage people live in the present—they enjoy the moment. Just as the lack of forgiveness can spoil the present, so can negative anticipation of the future, or worry. Vintage People have learned to worry less about the future. At first, I didn't

177

really understand this philosophy. After all, Vintage People have had a lot of unforeseen things happen to them in their lives. On the surface, it seems that they should be the most paranoid about the future. They have fewer days left upon this earth, and death is looming out there somewhere, closer than it had been in youth.

The comedian Jerry Seinfeld has a routine where he talks about older people driving. He says that he feels older people ought to have a higher speed limit, since they have less time left. As you get older, according to his theory, you should be allowed to drive faster. And once you reach one hundred, you should be allowed to go as fast as you want!

Of course, that's not the case. In spite of fewer days left on earth Vintage People seem to slow down, settle back, and worry less about the future. Even after seeing all the adversities that life can bring, they are at peace. My own theory is that Vintage People actually become this way *because of* the hardships they have experienced. They realize their physical being is becoming more fragile as they age. They become hardened or seasoned with the years and accept the things that come their way. They have also learned ways to enjoy the present while making the future seem a less scary place.

Vintage People have discovered a "coping mechanism" that psychologists often use to get people through troubled times. This is the "one day at a time" principle. I learned this survival technique in mid life when I found myself going through a divorce, working at a job I really didn't like, not seeing my children nearly as much as I wanted, and then suffering the loss of my oldest son in a car wreck when he was only seventeen. The only way I survived was to deliberately concentrate on living just one day at a time. I realized that at each moment, I was okay.

An old gospel song describes this philosophy. The words go like this:

One day at a time, sweet Jesus,
That's all I'm asking from you,
Just give me the strength to do every day what I
have to do.
Yesterday's gone, sweet Jesus, and tomorrow may
never be mine;
Lord help me today, show me the way, one day at a
time."

This view of life has helped a lot of people through troubled times. But Vintage People have found it to be a good philosophy of living all the time. What great joy comes with being able to enjoy the things of the moment. I've seen people who can't enjoy what's going on now because they are worried about the future. I remember one new mother I visited the day after the birth of her beautiful, healthy new son. This should have been one of the most ecstatic days of her life. But she was worried how the baby's older sister was going to accept him, when they could visit her parents (the weather was bad), and what they were going to do when he got older because they only had a two-bedroom house. Listening to all of her concerns, she began to make me anxious as well! During my short post delivery visit, she also expressed concern about not having enough "boy" clothes and even mentioned that she wasn't sure she knew how to potty train a boy! Worrying about the future was ruining the joy of the present.

Finally I had to interrupt this negative train of thought. "Wait a minute," I said. "You're getting way ahead of yourself. These things will all work out. Right now you should just savor the moment and enjoy the quiet time here in the hospital with your new son. This moment will never happen again, and you need to enjoy it while you can."

She wasn't able to completely get all the worries out of her mind, but she told me later that after I left, she just sat there, holding her baby, bonding with him, and enjoying the moment. "That's a time I will always remember and cherish," she said. "Thank you for reminding me to not overlook it."

She had taken one step towards becoming a Vintage Person. Vintage People don't worry about the future, but they plan for it. Planning is positive, worrying is negative. Studies of people of all ages show that most of the things we worry about never happen. Think about that. In some studies researchers have found that as much as ninety percent of the things one worries about never happen. The other ten percent that do happen are things that you generally have no control over anyway. They would have happened whether we worry about them or not. In most instances worrying about something does not change the outcome in any way. What a lot of energy we have used in the worrying process. We neglect enjoying the sunshine, people around us, our children, the flowers along the driveway, the robin's song, the company of our spouse, or the satisfactions that come at work, all because we are worrying about the future. Worrying about the future takes the joy out of the present.

I'm not saying that we should not think about the future. We all realize that if we spend our savings today we will have nothing to live on tomorrow. If we quit our jobs because we want to stay home to "enjoy the moment" we might not be able to eat tomorrow. But instead of worrying about the future, the positive approach is to plan for the future. Planning is a positive activity. Planning makes us feel better about the future, whereas worrying makes us feel worse. Planning does not stop you from being able to "enjoy the moment." As a matter of fact, planning frees you up to enjoy the moment even more.

There is a lot of fun in planning a vacation trip or for a dream home or the perfect dinner party. There is a sense of relief or satisfaction that comes from finally getting your

"Last Will and Testament" written. All of these things could be laden with a lot of worry. But planning takes the worry out of it. If we plan for most circumstances, then we don't need to worry about them. Planning is an activity done in the present to make the future less threatening.

One topic I heard about over and over when I interviewed Vintage People bothered me at first, but now I understand that it comes under the umbrella of planning so that worrying is not necessary. I found that a large number of Vintage People have already purchased their cemetery plots. Many have also pre-paid their own funerals. On the surface, this appears pessimistic, but now I know that was my hang-up and not theirs. They were comfortable with the idea. That part of the inevitable was already taken care of through planning, and now they were free to enjoy each remaining moment of their lives. What a valuable lesson for all of us to consider.

Now is the only time we have

In seminars I have attended about life-styles and quality of life, a popular exercise is to have all the participants write down the things you would do if you found out you had only six months to live—or three months, or twenty-four hours. Most people write a noble list including spending more time with loved ones, helping others and being benevolent. Some say they would quit their jobs and "smell the roses." Some would travel and see the world. Others would attempt to fulfill their dreams as quickly as possible.

These activities are the ideals of our lives. These are the things we really, truly, want to do with our lives. These are things that are important to us. We would not put them off if we knew we were running out of time. We would then truly be living in the moment. Some people say they would keep on working just as they are because they enjoy it. But no one writes down that they would try to earn more money, buy more cars, build a bigger house, or spend more time doing things they dislike.

After that list is finished, everyone is asked to make a list of what they are doing now. Most of these lists include working hard to make more money, buying more cars, building a bigger house, and doing a lot of things we really don't like doing! The two lists can then be compared. The concept is that the distance between what you are doing now and the ideal list of what you would do if you knew you had a very limited life left, indicates the level of stress in your life.

I think that is a good exercise, but there are some obvious flaws. I found a major one when I tried to do this with teenagers one time. They all listed "quit school" on their ideal list. Of course that is not consistent with a good future. But I think I probably agreed that if I had only a semester to live, I probably would not spent it studying calculus at the University of Kansas. Similarly, with just a few months to live, we could quit our jobs. But if we happen to live longer, we would be in trouble. Obviously, there was a major flaw in this study.

Does enjoying the moment mean that we have to spend our savings, throw caution to the wind, sell all our stocks, and have nothing left for the future? Is it reasonable to live each day as if there is no future? Is that what these exercises are supposed to teach us? I don't think so. The purpose of such activities is to help get the priorities of your life in line. Enjoying the moment is not inconsistent with looking ahead to the future or back to the past. Vintage People have learned to do both. Out of necessity, we all do things we don't want to do, but we must also realize that our life is NOW. Don't waste it! Enjoy each moment as fully as possible. We do have a limited amount of time on this planet.

A seventy-seven-year-old Vintage Minister told me this story that happened to him in his early ministry. He was ministering to a small congregation in a remote farm town in Kansas, over fifty years ago. Tragedy struck when a young farmer's wife in the congregation died following childbirth (which was far too common at that time). The farmer was left with three small children to raise.

The minister performed the funeral services, which of course, the farmer attended. However, on his way home from the funeral, the widowed farmer stopped at the home of his late wife's sister—and asked her to marry him!

She was shocked and replied: "Absolutely not! It hasn't been time yet. You just buried your wife!"

To this he responded: "Well, I've got a farm to work and three young children to take care of. I need a wife! If you won't marry me, I'm going on down to Mable's house and ask her. And if she won't, then I will keep going until I find someone who will!"

His former sister-in-law then responded: "Well, I guess if that's the case, then I better marry you!"

The minister married the couple two weeks later, and they were happy together for forty-five years, until the farmer died!

True story! This farmer was living his life in the present. He was not dwelling on the past. He wasn't sure of his future, but he knew what he needed right then. He didn't stop and worry about what the neighbors would think or what society considered proper. He was living in the moment. This is another characteristic that Vintage People seem to have learned.

In contrast to this story, I have a patient who lost her husband of thirty-two years. An old friend whose wife had recently divorced him for a delivery man, called to comfort her. One thing led to another and after six months he asked her to marry him. She refused because of "what will people think?" They put off their happiness for two years until she felt the time was finally right. Then, two weeks after they were married, he had a heart attack and died! She told me later: "I don't know why I waited. Who cares what other people think! We could have had almost two years of happiness before he was taken away."

Vintage People have learned that the past is gone. Nor is there life later down the road. The future may never come, but the present is ours to live as fully as we can. This is where Vintage People have the advantage. Through experience and maturity, they have learned to "enjoy the moment." They live the days they have left and draw power from them. We all have that choice. Why wait until it looks right to the neighbors?

Risk

Several years ago there was a story of a reporter for a sports magazine who came up with a gimmick. He thought it would be interesting to take one of America's popular football quarterback heroes of the time out to Jack London's grave, and get a "dumb jock's" reaction to some of the world's greatest classical poetry ever written. He finally was able to arrange such an interview. The reporter and the quarterback went to Jack London's grave, and the reporter read the following quote:

> "I'd rather be ashes than dust, I'd rather my spark go
> out in a burning flame than it be stifled with dry rot.
> I'd rather be a splendid meteor blazing across the
> sky, every atom in me in magnificent glow, than to
> be a sleepy and permanent planet. Life is to be
> lived—not exist. I shall not waste my days trying to
> prolong them. I will use my time!"

I love that quote and believe that it describes how Vintage People live. Back to the story. The reporter then turned to what he thought was a dumb athlete and asked, "Now, as an athlete, what does this quote mean to you?"

The quarterback put his thumbs inside his belt loops, looked down at the ground and kicked at the dirt. He thought a moment, bit his lower lip, and then said, "Throw deep!"

Vintage People throw deep in life. They go for all the marbles; they go for broke; every atom in magnificent glow!

Vintage People are risk takers, but they take safe risks. There is a big difference between being reckless and in taking safe risks. In the history books General George S. Patton, who spearheaded the Allied victory over Nazi Germany, is depicted as an impetuous risk taker on the battlefield. However, on D-Day, the sixth of June 1944, Patton wrote in a letter to his son, a West Point cadet, "Take calculated risks. That is far from being rash."

That sentence with its plea for good judgment helps explain the real reason that Patton was so successful on the battlefield. Although he was decisive and quick to act, he looked before he leaped. He knew what he was getting into. He took risks but used judgment.

Through mistakes as well as successes, Vintage People have learned what risks are worth taking. Herein lies power. They have learned that anything worthwhile in life involves some risk. As Will Rogers said, "You've got to go out on a limb sometimes, because that's where the fruit is!" Vintage People tell me they have gotten where they are only by taking calculated risks. This involves all areas of their lives including business, personal life, and even relationships. Their philosophy seems to be, "You never know until you try!"

One wealthy and successful retired investment broker I know told me this story: "I was giving a class at a nearby town on investments. One young man in the back of the room kept questioning everything I advised. He was beginning to really annoy me. Finally after I had made what I thought was a very good presentation on a particular investment strategy he said: 'I just can't believe you would take that kind of risk!' "

"I had taken all I could from him," he continued. "And I am very proud of my reply. I said: 'If you are afraid of that risk, that's why I am teaching this course, and you are taking it!' He didn't bother me the rest of the evening!"

An eighty-one-year-old nurse wrote: "When I look back upon my life I have always felt I will regret more the things I failed to do than the things I tried and failed." This remarkable lady joined the Peace Corps in her early sixties and climbed Mt. Kenya (17,500 ft.) when she was sixty-three. On a recent summer, at eighty-one years of age, she traveled back to Kenya with a Japanese volunteer that she had known earlier in the Peace Corps and helped set up emergency medical clinics.

Think about it. What is the worst thing that can happen if you take a risk? You fail. Vintage People don't see failure as a negative thing. They see it as a learning experience. Many told me they had learned far more from their failures than from their successes. Failure seems stimulating to them. In fact, researchers who study what helps keep our minds young and functioning say that failing and putting ourselves in difficult positions often is accompanied by significant growth. One Vintage Lady wrote, "I think the biggest risk in life would be to take no risks at all!"

I love the story about Wayne Gretzky, the leading scorer in the history of ice hockey. Early in his career he was often hesitant to take shots at the goal. When his coach asked him about that, he explained that he was afraid of missing and bringing down his average score. To this, his coach is said to have replied; "Wayne, you miss one hundred percent of the shots you never take!" He began to take more shots, and the rest is history.

The truly Vintage People I know seem to live by this rule. A retired Air Force Pilot told me, "If you take safe risks, and it turns out wrong, you can do several things about it. You can try to change it and make it right if possible. Best of all, you can learn from it. If you just can't learn from it, then you may need to just forget it and go on with your life." Then he added with a chuckle, "If nothing else works you can always lie and deny you did it!"

Once you have missed out on something, it may be gone forever. Opportunities often sprint across our lives like a rabbit running for cover. If we wait to take advantage of them, they never re-appear. When I think about my life, most of my significant opportunities have had very narrow windows. If I hadn't gone to college when I did, I probably would not have gone later. If I had not gone to medical school when I did, I certainly never would have had the chance later in life. Having children, attending a certain college class that changed my life, even asking my wife for that first date, are all opportunities that could have been easily missed. Vintage People try to keep their list of missed opportunities as short as possible.

Vintage People accept the fact that risk implies possible failure. They are careful that benefits to be gained from taking the risk and winning outweigh the possible ill effects of losing. They know when to push on and when to stop. There are situations where persistence pays off. When Thomas Edison was doing experiment after experiment searching for the perfect filament for the incandescent light bulb, his co-workers tended to get discouraged. "Shucks," he told one such assistant, "we haven't failed. We now know a thousand things that won't work, so we're that much closer to finding what will."

In some situations it makes sense to stop and put your energy elsewhere. If a business venture, project, or personal relationship continues to fail, do we persist until we are financially or emotionally bankrupt? This is were Vintage People excel. They seem to know when to be persistent, but also when to stop. They know when to quit, learn from an experience, and then move on. One Vintage gentleman told me: "Several years ago I read a quote from W. C. Fields which says, 'If at first you don't succeed, try again. If the second time you still do not succeed, try once again. But if the third time you do not succeed, quit! There's no use being a fool about it!' That saying has served me well in my life."

Younger people often take foolish risks with their health, with their finances, and even with their lives. They take risks without much chance of significant reward. Risking your life to drive one hundred miles per hour, to beat that train to the crossing to save five minutes of your day, or to risk your entire future by dropping out of school when the going gets tough, doesn't make sense to the Vintage Person. They measure the risk against the possible benefits. This requires judgment that comes with maturity and experience.

A Latin proverb says, "A ship in harbor is safe, but that's not why ships were built." That's not why humans were built, either. Jesus describes the importance of safe risks to us in His parable of the talents. A landowner traveled to Rome, and while he was gone, left each of three servants with sums of money. While the owner was gone, two of the servants invested the money, bargained, and took some safe risks. They were able to double their master's money. However, the third servant "was afraid." He took the money and buried it in the ground. He took no risk. But at the same time, there was no chance of any gain either. Even though the third servant still had the same amount of money when his master returned, the landowner was upset.

"You should at least have put my money into the bank so I could have some interest," he said.

Then the landowner took the money from the third servant and gave it to the servant who has made the most money. At the end, Jesus explains the parable by saying, "For the man who uses well what he is given shall be given more, and he shall have abundance."

Vintage People never bury their money or their talents. They see life as something to be lived. By taking safe risks, their lives become richer, and they gain from those who do not risk. Somehow, through maturity Vintage People have developed a sense for which risks are worth taking and which will be rewarding. They know when to throw deep! What a wonderful characteristic to be harvested by the rest of us!

Hope

Vintage People have learned that they can enjoy the moment more when they have hope for the future. Living in the present is important, but living in the moment by itself is very shallow. My two dogs do that. They are large, outside farm dogs who are happy all the time. They live in the moment. They get up each morning, chase squirrels, dig in the garden, and lie in the sun. They eat when fed and give no thought to what the future may bring. They never save anything or plan for the future. They are successful as dogs but not very successful in business, or in life. They don't own their own home, have a color television, or even buy their own food. They contribute to the universe only by pleasing the humans around them, and they could not live without us. They don't have productive jobs, raise children, go to church, or read books. They don't teach the next generation of dogs. But they are happy—enjoying the moment.

Likewise, small children have very little concept of the future. An hour is like a year to a three-year-old. They are interested only in immediate gratification and what will please them at the moment. It's in the teen-age years that the sense of future with hopes and dreams begins to flicker. Of course at that age teenagers feel themselves invincible, but at least they are beginning to dream and set goals for the future.

Hope, which contains dreams and goals, is a strictly human characteristic. No other species has hope. It is extremely important to our happiness, our health, and our success. Saint Paul was aware of this when he wrote to the Romans, "...we rejoice in our sufferings, knowing that suffering produces endurance, and endurance produces character, and character produces hope, and hope does not disappoint us..."

It may seem inconsistent for me to include a section on hope in the chapter on "enjoying the moment." After all, living in the moment involves the present. Hope, with dreams and goals, involves the future. Didn't we just say that Vintage People have learned how to live in the present? Can they also live in the future at the same time? I've found that this is exactly what they do. Vintage People have discovered that hope, goals, and dreams—in the future—actually enhance their lives in the present. John Maxwell says, "If there is hope in your future, there is power in your present!" This is a powerful statement, and I hope I can explain what it means.

Dealing with patients I have found one of the greatest medicines is hope. Without hope people feel no reason to live, no reason to go on. With hope things are accomplished which we may view as miraculous. I think we do a great dis-service if we take someone's hope away, whether we are a parent, a friend, a teacher, a boss, or a physician. No one should let anyone or anything take away their hope for the future.

I have seen what can happen to patients when someone takes away their hope. This is one of the major objections I have with permanent disability determinations. Once you are labeled as having a certain percentage of disability, that label never goes away. Even worse, in my opinion, is the practice some physicians have of predicting life expectancy based on a diagnosis. I violently object to the traditional statements that patients and families of supposedly dying patients have been told for years, such as "You have six months to live!" What does that do but destroy all hope? And the way the human mind works, if a knowledgeable authority makes a statement like that, then it may come true.

I have been astonished at how this principle of the human mind has worked to my benefit in my practice of obstetrics. The most common question I am asked by women in labor and their families is, "When will the baby be born?" Without thinking too much about it, I gave them a time—like two o'clock. It was an educated guess, but I was surprised at how often I was right! I started feeling pretty smug about my forecasts, and the nurses began to plan around my predictions. My wife even started to plan meals around my predictions.

My bubble burst, however, when I figured out what was really happening. The mind of a patient in this condition is extremely open to suggestion. When I, as an experienced doctor, gave them a specific time of delivery, their minds interpreted it as fact. They expected to have their baby at a certain time. As long as the prediction was reasonable, the contracting muscles and the patient's interpretation of when to start pushing the baby out all strove for that goal! Often, the patients would tell me, "I felt like pushing at nine-thirty, just like you told me I would!"

I've not admitted to the nursing staff or to my wife what is really happening here. I prefer to let them think I am just good. But in my own mind I realize it is the power of the human mind that is making my predictions accurate. It is a principle of hope, of expectation, and of having a goal.

In predicting times of birth, I don't think I am doing any harm. If I use this same power of the human mind to take away someone's hope and predict a limited life expectancy, however, it is a tragedy. Whenever physicians tell patients what they can't do in a negative way, they limit that patient's potential. Happily, we are learning not to do that.

Most physicians can tell anecdotes where medical predictions were wrong and hope has prevailed. About six years ago I met Helen, seventy-six years old. She had come to my office for a complete physical exam. Visiting with her I found that she had not seen a physician for years. I also learned that her husband had died a number of years before, but she had recently met a wonderful gentleman. They were planning to get married soon, and she seemed to glow with happiness. She admitted that she felt "like a schoolgirl!"

For the first time in years, she said she felt like she had something to live for. She was full of hope and dreams. That is what had prompted her to come in for the physical exam. I did the usual exam for her age, including a Pap smear, since she had not had one in years. Everything seemed fine and I reassured her as she left the office.

About three days later the pathologist called me to get more information about her Pap smear. It was a busy afternoon, and my heart sank as he told me, "the smear is packed with malignant appearing endometrial cells!" In English, this means the patient had cancer of the uterus and it was spilling out to where I was able to collect some of the cells on the Pap smear—obviously a bad sign. It was Friday afternoon, and I just didn't want to call her with that kind of news before the weekend, since we couldn't do anything until Monday anyway.

Monday morning I began trying to reach her. Finally, my nurse was able to track down her daughter who got a message to Helen that night. She had been out shopping for her wedding dress all day. She finally came into the office the next day at my request. I explained the situation to her and recommended that she let me refer her to a specialist right away. I thought she understood and that I had adequately stressed the seriousness of the disease. But to my surprise, she didn't seem concerned. She replied, "I really don't have time for that right now. I'm getting married next week, and I'm not letting anything interfere with that! I'll be back after my honeymoon!"

Exactly five weeks later she returned and said that she and her husband had discussed it, and she was ready to see the specialist now. Of course, surgery was recommended. A hysterectomy was done, but at the time of the surgery, the surgeon reported metastatic disease to the ligaments and other structures in the pelvis. He was unable to remove all the small tumors. The pathology report confirmed endometrial cancer with all the lymph nodes removed being positive for cancer. But, Helen refused chemotherapy or radiation, and was therefore sent back to me to "talk some sense into" her!

This time her husband was with her. I had not met him before, but he was a robust appearing man, who looked younger than his age. They were holding hands in the exam room, and both seemed happy. It was only three weeks after her surgery, but she appeared very well. Her first question to me was, "When can I drive the car again?" The second question was, "How long before Sam and I can make love again?" Obviously, they were not dwelling on the cancer.

Finally I was able to approach the topic of the pathology report and the fact that she still had cancer. I remember her response very well. "Doc," she started out, "I'm happier than I have been in years. I have hope. Sam and I have lots of dreams. Doctors told my mother she had cancer, and she never went back! Mom lived a long life and finally died of a heart attack about twenty years later. I expect that will happen to me, too."

At last I understood her reasoning. She not only had hope for the future, but she had an expectation from what had happened to her mother. She was happy, she had love in her life, and she had a goal of living long and not dying from cancer, just like her mother. I remember thinking to myself, "Well, she's happy! She might just as well live the days that she has left without all the discomfort of radiation and chemotherapy. After all, I can't make her do something against her will. My job is to advise her medically, and I've done that."

From the medical information available to me, I would have expected to see her again in less that six months for pain control and terminal care. Time went on and I kind of forgot about Helen, until I saw her and her husband in the grocery store about nine months later. They were still holding hands. They recognized me and spoke. When I asked how she was the reply was, "I've never felt better! Sam and I really appreciate all that you have done. I'll be back to see you if I ever need a doctor again!"

That was over five years ago. I recently spoke to a Christian Women's Club meeting, and Helen was on the front row, looking as happy as ever, at eighty-one years of age. If she is sick, she doesn't know it! My theory is that she has so much hope and is so happy that the cancer doesn't have a chance. She is just ignoring it and living her life with the expectation that she will die in her nineties from a heart attack like her mother did. Someday I will probably find out—if I'm still alive!

There is always hope. It's an old statement, and the origin has been lost, but it's true. "Where there is life, there is hope." Helen is living proof of that.

As we age, it is important to hold onto that kind of hope, the kind of hope that Helen has. As we become Vintage People our goals will change, but hope must always be present. I remember a time in my own life where I felt I had accomplished all my goals. I had a successful medical practice, a nice family, and we had built our dream home. Suddenly, life seemed stagnant! I had no goals or dreams. Hope was gone. The fun was gone. That is an unfortunate thing to happen. Guard against it.

If you have ever planned for a very special goal, you probably remember that half of the fun was in the planning and the anticipation. Just having the goal and the hope of accomplishing that goal is invigorating. Vintage People realize that if they accomplish one goal, they must set up others. I have found that as people age, their goals usually become less material and more altruistic. The joy received from volunteer work in the hospital, in public service organizations, in churches, and even in business becomes more important than making money. Money seems less important than service. Without hope and purpose, life doesn't have quality. Vintage People don't let that happen. Successful aging means continuing to have goals and hope of accomplishing those goals.

Statistics about legal immigrants who come to this country are revealing. A legal immigrant coming to the United States has four times the chance of becoming a millionaire than you or I who are born here. Think about it!

These people give up their language, their culture, their possessions, relatives and family members to come here. What is the one thing that they have? Hope. A dream! A goal! Many times they accomplish that dream or that goal before they find out it can't be done. Think of what we could do with that same kind of hope and that same dream!

Our medical clinic interviewed a prospective physician with an amazing story. He had been a physician in Argentina. But he left to come here to the United States and worked in a car wash until he could get into a residency program. He would rather work in a car wash in this country than to be a physician in Argentina. He was motivated by hope. He was willing to give up all that he had to follow his dream for the future.

Most great leaders are motivated by hope. Martin Luther King Jr. had a dream. The founders of the constitution had a dream. Thomas Edison had hope. That one characteristic, probably above all others, helped them to be successful in their goals.

All great buildings, all roadway networks, the space shuttle, modern medical techniques—all great enterprises—started out as someone's dream that involved hope for the future. If we were living just in the present, we would not reach out to the future with projects that take several years to complete. Vintage People, with their experience of accumulated years know this and seem to enjoy the present much more, because the future exists.

TWELVE

FRIENDS

"He who has a thousand friends has not a friend to
spare."
—Omar Khayyam

My friends are the most important thing I have," writes
a ninety-two-year-old Vintage Lady. "I know I could not
have lived this long, or been this successful without my dear
friends." Vintage People have learned how to get along with
people and how to have friends. They know there is power
in friendships. One of their major characteristics that allows
them to become Vintage People is knowing how to make
and keep friends. They enjoy having friends around. Not
many people fulfill their potential as humans without
friends.

As I have gotten to know Vintage People, I have been
struck by the depth and magnitude of their friendships. They
have built love and friendship into their lives. Vintage People have discovered that they are less depressed and less
withdrawn when they are socializing with their friends. I
was astonished to find the diversity of the friendships that
Vintage People maintain. Young and old, men and women,
people of all walks of life—all seem to be in the friendship
circle. Vintage People seem to have learned that life's
defeats are easier to take when we they have people around
for support. We all need to keep friendships in repair and to
make new friends to replace those that drift away from time
to time.

Be a friend

Not only have Vintage People learned how to get along with
people and how to have friends, but they have also learned
how to *be* a friend. This is one of their primary characteristics of successful living. In analyzing all the suggestions and
all the various tips they have given me about forming
friendships, I think it all boils down to what modern psychologists call the "Law of Indirect Effort." This mental law
was discussed in Chapter Four when we considered self-
esteem, but it also applies to friendships. To review, this
principle says that we often get what we want by giving
away what we want.

In friendships we frequently get what we want in an
indirect way. What we put into the friendship is what we get
back. In other words, to have a friend, we must be a friend.

This Law of Indirect Effort works in all aspects of
friendship and human relations. If we want someone to like
us, we have to like them. If we want to impress someone,
the best way to do that is to be impressed by them! If we
want someone to believe in us, than we have to believe in
them. If we want someone to help us, help them first. The
best way to have someone interested in us, is to be interested in them. In *Roads to Radiant Living*, Charles L. Allen
says, "You can make more friends in a month by being
interested in them than in ten years by trying to get them
interested in you." Norman Vincent Peale says simply,
"Getting people to like you is only the other side of liking
them."

What a powerful canon for living! These rules can be
applied to almost any situation in human relationships. And
they work! Love your spouse, and he or she will love you.
Respect your children, and there's a good chance they will
respect you. Be interested in your friends, and they will be
interested in you. Think about what you did when you were

dating. If there was a girl or guy you happened to like, you tried to learn as much as you could about what the person liked. Talking about what your potential friend liked got you more points than always talking about what you liked. (Some people have never learned this principle!) Salespersons make a lot of money by focusing on what the client wants and what the client's interests are. Sincerity weighs in heavily here. People pick up on insincere remarks rapidly.

As a corollary to "being a friend," Vintage People have also learned the value of forming varied friendships. Experts in modern psychology tell us that people have a "healthy personality" to the same degree that they get along with a diverse group of people. Successful Vintage People usually have friends of different races, religious backgrounds, and ages. It means having friends of the opposite sex. It might even mean being friends with your business competitors. It means learning from and enjoying people who are different from you.

I've seen the opposite happen so many times in my practice of medicine with negative, depressed housewives. They seem to form friendships only with other negative, depressed housewives. They get together basically because they hate the same people and the same things about their dull lives. They dislike everyone else who is different from them and are jealous of anyone who is happy. They share morning coffee, and compete to see whose life is worse. All these narrow friendships do is make their dull lives duller and more negative, and drive them further into depression!

I'm usually not able to convince these people to break the cycle, because if I don't agree with them, then I am not their friend. Still, it is a great principle of life that those with the healthiest personalities—the happiest people—are able to get along with the most diverse group of friends. Those who cannot get along with anyone else have the lowest self-esteem, and the poorest personalities of all. Most of the people at that end of the spectrum live their lives in a miserable existence.

Again, the Bible, the greatest book of human psychology ever written, emphasizes this point. "If you love only those who love you, what credit is that to you? For sinners, too, love those who love them. And if you treat well those who treat you well, what credit is that to you?...But love your enemies; do good and lend without prospect of return. Then your return will be rich." (Luke 6:32-35, Modern Language Version)

Another skill that Vintage People seem to master is how to treat people the way those people want to be treated. People with a poor personality try only one method of interacting in social relations. If that method doesn't work, they just do the same thing harder. They treat everyone the same way. Successful Vintage People have more than one personality skill. They treat different people differently and are keen judges as to how to treat various people. If one approach doesn't work, they have other approaches to try.

Vintage People have learned the great principles of friendship but also recognize the values of friendship itself. As one Vintage Gentleman told me with a sly smile, "I think friends are very important. You need at least six of them when you die! Wouldn't it be awful if one of the handles on the coffin were open!"

Best friends

Recently I had the privilege of hearing a successful Vintage attorney, business man, and state senator, deliver an address. At the conclusion of his speech he gave one bit of advice about how to be truly successful in life. "Find someone who is smarter, and more talented than you are—and marry her!

Then, be each other's best friends for the rest of your life. That is one of the wisest career choices you can make!"

"I was so lucky," states one ninety-year-old Vintage Lady. "I was married to my best friend for sixty-four years." I can personally affirm that life is wonderful when you are married to your best friend. A couple I know confirmed this feeling. The wife said, "I can't think of anything I would rather do with someone else other than my husband— except shopping! I'd rather shop with my sister!" Both of them agreed on that.

But men and women are different! Yet most of us, including Vintage People, spend nearly all of our adult lives living with someone of the opposite sex. How do we do it? We have physical differences and psychological differences. Our brains work differently. It is a proven fact that women have more trouble with directions and reading maps than men do. Men have more problems picking up on emotions, and are totally lost trying to figure out feelings.

Scientists have always suspected that men and women think differently. For years, experts have tried to find ana- tomical differences in the brains of men and women but have found only a few, and they seem to be insignificant. Anatomy seems to be much less important than function. However, recently, by using modern imaging techniques, researchers have noticed distinct changes in how the brain functions—how we think! We have totally different "soft- ware." Men and women have the same anatomical hardware in the brain, but we are programmed differently.

These differences start very early in childhood. Even without adult prompting, a little girl at play will daintily set up her dolls and tea set with all the little plastic cups and saucers. What does her brother do? He assembles his Legos into a monster truck and ambushes the tea party! Even as children we behave differently, and also develop differently.

Little girls develop language skills much quicker than their male counterparts. In studies I've seen in which researchers have attached a microphone to little girls and boys and followed them throughout the day, the average three-year-old girl will speak about 12,000 words. She doesn't need anyone to talk to—she will talk to herself, to her dolls, and sometimes to just nobody! Little boys speak fewer than half that many words.

So how is it, considering all these differences, that Vintage People are so good at living with their spouses? Statistics show us that the divorce rate is lower in the older age groups. At first I thought that "back then," somehow, everyone just happened to marry the "right person." But in my interviews I found that many Vintage People had not really had the opportunity to search for the "right" person. Many married the "girl or boy next door." Many had never dated more than one or two people. One Vintage Couple had a pre-arranged marriage set up by their parents—and they have been together sixty-three years. It appears there are other factors involved here besides just finding the right person.

Another possibility is that economic factors kept them together, as many women prior to our current generation were not employed and would find it hard to support themselves if not married. Society several decades ago was not nearly as accepting of divorce as it is today. Male and female roles were more defined and accepted by each partner. Also, perhaps Vintage People are a product of times when expectations were not so high. Times were rough, and people accepted the rough times in their marriages as well.

Somehow they made marriage work. I'm not saying that there are no single or divorced Vintage People. Some are unhappy and probably should be divorced, but most Vintage People have at some time in their lives maintained a long-term marital relationship. Many of the characteristics that help Vintage People make, and be, good friends also helps in marriage. Accepting your spouse for whoever he or she is comes first. Building up your spouse helps your own self-esteem. When you build someone else up, by the Law of Indirect Effort you build yourself up too. There are all kinds of little things that spouses can do to continually support and build each other up and keep each other happy.

Talking with Vintage People, I have discovered wisdom about relationships. Most relationships start with "chemistry"—that mysterious force that seems to attract us to certain individuals and not others. Science has yet to figure that one out. But a successful marriage is based on more than that. All that "chemistry" does is narrow down the field of possible mates. From the lack of "chemistry" we can eliminate about 99 percent of the population of the opposite sex that we do not want to consider living with! Of those few where the "chemistry" is right, you have to explore all the other factors: likes and dislikes, things that you have in common, moral values, ambitions in life, religious beliefs, and general temperament. The list goes on and on. When we look at all these factors, it is amazing that anyone ever marries the "right" person. I'm not sure that they do. Most Vintage People tell me that instead of making the right decision, they made their decision "right!" That is, once they were married, they proceeded as if they would always be husband and wife and never looked back.

Psychologists tell us that the more things we have in common with our mate, the more compatible we will be. Opposites attract only in temperament. For example, someone who is shy may be attracted to someone who is outgoing because they can complement each other. In all other things from food to movies to the brand of car to drive, the more we have in common, the better for our relationship.

Many Vintage People had a lot in common with their spouse when they married—because neither one had anything! It was hard to argue over which brand of cornflakes to buy when there was only one brand available. You had to agree on your favorite color of car, when they all came in black! Vintage People developed their tastes together. One Vintage lady told me, "We didn't have much when we married—just each other. But one of my favorite memories is of lying on the floor—no furniture—holding each other!" They are now rather affluent, but have grown and developed together.

In our world today there are certainly a lot more areas of possible conflict because there is so much more variety and availability. A couple in my practice almost didn't get married because they couldn't agree on whether to spend their honeymoon in Europe or the Bahamas. Most Vintage People didn't have to make those kinds of choices, because they could afford neither option!

Vintage People also tend to bring into their marriages the knowledge that they are human, and that their spouse is human as well. They will both make mistakes. In dealing with patients going through divorce, and having been there personally, I think this is where so many couples fail. If you expect your spouse to be perfect and withhold love when they are not, the seeds are planted for disaster. If our mates cannot accept our failures and flaws and harp on our faults because they want us to change or improve, guilt and depression are generated. Enough guilt and a person will feel unlovable. And when the situation becomes too painful to bear, the person will find a way out of the relationship.

The most amazing thing I learned about the marriages of Vintage People was that they learned how to use the differences between men and women to their advantage. They learned to draw upon the strengths of each other. For most, this was not a conscious effort, but it evolved as they lived their lives together. And "together" was a key. Almost all the Vintage People I know make it a habit of discussing all major decisions with each other. They are truly best friends. They respect one another's opinions. There is nothing they cannot discuss together. Husbands and wives are involved in each other's lives, which prevents them from ever growing apart. Wives know what is happening in their husband's business, and husbands know what happens where their wives work and at home. They share information back and forth. Perhaps the wife can give her husband insight from her more sensitive perspective, into some of the problems he is dealing with at work. Maybe the husband can give practical advice in the decisions his wife has to make. This draws upon the richness of both male and female. It is here that a couple's power is greater than the sum of the power of two individuals.

One last comment about this subject, from a wise retired minister concerning males and females: "Women, I hope you find all the freedoms you want. But don't become men. God has given you some very special gifts for nurturing humanity that men don't have. Don't lose those. And men, don't be grudging of women you know. God has also given you talents to see things differently than they do. The world needs both of these perspectives. We are not competitors in life, but are to use our special skills to help each other."

That seems to be how Vintage People have approached the relationships with their spouses. And it works. Whatever the reason, long term marital relationships are a characteristic of Vintage People. They have found there is power to be successful when your spouse is your best friend. And most all Vintage People I have interviewed say they have been either "happy," or "very happy" in their union. After all, in Genesis, it was God Himself who said, "It is not good that the man should be alone; I will make him a helper fit for him."

Be a friend to a child

Among the friendships that Vintage People savor are the friendships of children. Something about talking to a child refreshes the spirit and renews our soul. Jesus said, "Suffer the little children to come unto me, and forbid them not; for of such is the kingdom of God." Children seem closer to heaven than any other creatures with whom we can have dialogue. They enter this world carrying some of that radiant glow that lifts the spirits of all those around them. It is hard to remain sad, angry or depressed for long when you are talking to a child.

I once observed small children playing after the funeral of an uncle of mine. It was their great uncle who had died, and their great aunt was still crying as we returned home after the funeral. But within a few minutes, the children began to fight over who got to sit on her lap. They were extremely honest and asked her why she was crying, since Uncle Wilburn was now with God. They began to ask other questions, and within fifteen minutes, the widow was up and fixing them Kool-Aid. They were laughing and by their actions appeared to be saying that life goes on. My aunt seemed to realize that as long as there are young lives to nurture, she, too, must go on.

Vintage People have discovered the benefits of being energized by small children. They look forward to seeing their grandchildren and often visit with children at church or in the neighborhood. One Vintage lady tells me that "...a hug and a 'I love you grandma,' from her five-year-old granddaughter, is better than Prozac!"

Why do children have this effect? I think it is because children have many of the same characteristics of Vintage People, and that these are traits we all admire. For one thing, kids are completely honest. One grandmother put it this way, "I can be confident that little children never make up things that I say. But they often repeat word for word what I never should have said in the first place!"

I will never forget my two-year-old cousin walking over to his neighbor's yard while she was doing yard work. A thin person, she stopped pulling weeds to visit with him. As my aunt was walking over to be sure he was all right, she saw my little cousin lean back, put his hands on his hips and look the lanky neighbor straight in the eye as he proclaimed, "My Daddy calls you 'Old Buzzard Bait!' " Kids are honest!

Children also have an enthusiasm and exuberance for life that is contagious. They see life as new and exciting. Everything fascinates them, from the dead bug on the side-walk to the special rock they carry in their pocket. They help remind Vintage People where they have been and what is really important in life. Once all the hurry and worry and pressure of making a living and solving all the adult prob-lems of the world is over, Vintage People like to know there is still a place where a simple caterpillar on a blade of grass is the highlight of someone's day. They like to see that someone still sees rainy days and mud puddles as things of joy to explore. It is refreshing to hear someone ask the same questions that adults are fearful to answer, such as "Who made God?" or "Why is the grass green?"

I think that by talking to a child we get a sense of "awe" about life and the universe. And we are reminded of the simple acceptance that we once knew ourselves.

Dr. Seuss says that "Adults are obsolete children." Perhaps grandchildren are God's way of showing us that we are not so obsolete after all. Vintage People have the maturity and wisdom to see life again from a child's eyes. They realize the cycle of beginning and ending, of birth and death, of renewal and stagnation.

Children are uninhibited when it comes to having fun. Play is something that is done just for fun— no other function. Adults need to remember how to play. As adults we have few activities left that are purely for fun. Even the things we call "play" are often highly competitive athletic events with each participant trying to win. And what about the relaxing round of golf? It often takes a nasty turn when we don't score the way we envision. These things are not truly "play." Children can teach us to have fun. Watch children at play with a cardboard box. They are not trying to accomplish anything, not competing with anyone; they are simply having fun. What a wonderful attribute for Vintage People, and all of us, to mimic.

"Every child is an artist," said Pablo Picasso. "The problem is how to remain an artist once he grows up." As adults, we lose some of the childish qualities of innocence, of curiosity, and of seeing life as exciting. Vintage People have discovered that they can draw strength from the companionship of these small containers of energy. Vintage People should always be able to look out the window and see children playing. It is a mistake, I think, to have retirement communities where children are not allowed. We have talked about the importance of having a diversity of friends. Children must be included in this variety. The purest friendship the heart can contain is the sincere love of a five-year-old.

George F. Will states it well. "Biologically, adults produce children. Spiritually, children produce adults. Most of us do not grow up until we have helped children do so. Thus do the generations form a braided cord."

Acquaintances

When I began interviewing Vintage People, I noticed that they commonly talked about their "friends." Almost every subject I approached, they had a friend who had been there, had done it, or knew how to get it done! I wondered to myself, "How could they have this many friends?" Slowly I began to realize that when they were talking of "friends," they were talking about what I would call acquaintances. Vintage People considered anyone who might recognize their face or know their name as a friend. Anyone they have ever met is a "friend." What a beautiful attitude! A retired pharmaceutical salesman I know explained it by saying, "Strangers are just friends that I haven't met yet!"

One obvious reason that Vintage People have so many friends is that they have lived longer—they have had more time to develop friendships. However, I suspect that if you factored their age into a formula that somehow compensated for the number of years they have lived, Vintage People would still have disproportionately more friends. They recognize the importance of "acquaintances" as well as close friends. They have learned how to cultivate friendship with peripheral acquaintances they often talk about.

I have also found that the pool of peripheral friends Vintage People possess is not limited necessarily to people who like them. They often include business rivals, political rivals, and sometimes even bitter enemies, in their definition of friends. Vintage People have identified some positive, likable trait that they can respect in almost everyone. Being able to find traits to respect in others is the first step

in making and keeping friends. This is a powerful characteristic for success.

What other characteristics do Vintage People have that
allows them to develop so many varied friends? I would put
several of these under the general heading of making other
people feel important. When I specifically asked Vintage
People about this, a huge number of them quoted me the
"Golden Rule"—treat other people the way you want to be
treated.

"Accept everyone as they are," advised an eighty-year-
old who considered himself a friend to everyone. "When
you pick a friend, you are accepting them warts and all—the
good and the bad. It's important not to judge."

"Smile," says another Vintage Lady. "That lets the person know you value them—even before you speak the first
words."

"I try to find something to compliment each new friend
on," says another. Sincere praise does seem to go a long
way. Vintage People have discovered how to make praise
effective. Psychologists agree that the more specific the
praise, the more beneficial it is. Just saying, "You are a great
person!" is not nearly as effective as saying, "I really like
the way you handled that situation." The sooner praise is
given after the praise-worthy event, the more effective it is.

It is easy to compliment women on their clothing, first
of all, because most women dress nicely. Secondly, most
women pick out their own clothes, so when you compliment
their clothing, you are giving them a personal compliment—you are saying that they have good taste. But what
about men? Most men wear black suits, and their wives usually pick those out. One trick I learned from a seminar
speaker was to look at men's neckties. That is usually the
only part of his wardrobe that he himself has selected. I
have never complimented a man on his necktie without get-

ting a satisfied smile and a big "thank you" in return. This has become a standing joke where I have spoken and told this story. It's not unusual after I have made my presentation for two hundred people to compliment me on my tie! Thankfulness is another key ingredient in developing acquaintances that never goes out of style. A salesman told me that he felt he could never say "thank you" too much. Many Vintage People have conquered the art of saying "thank you." Written notes, a phone call, and just a heartfelt "thanks" will win many friends. The value in giving the thank you is proportionate to the weight it carries to the receiver.

Many Vintage People have learned the uselessness of criticizing or arguing with potential friends. "No one likes to be wrong," says a wise Vintage Gentleman. "You just as well save your breath, and let them have their opinion—and you keep yours!"

Psychology has proven that human beings are rationalizing creatures. We can convince ourselves that we are right in almost any situation. Even the worst criminals can justify their actions and say they were right to do what they did under the circumstances. So we seldom get anywhere by criticizing or arguing with others. This principle especially applies to husbands and wives. Has anyone ever truly "won" an argument with his or her spouse? Vintage People know this. Unfortunately, you and I are just not going to be able to straighten someone else out, no matter how much we criticize or argue. As a matter of fact, when we criticize or argue, we usually cause the other person to dig in deeper and to be just that much more determined to prove us wrong. Most of us react that way when someone begins to criticize our opinion. Remember the law of indirect effort? When we criticize others, we tear ourselves down. As a wise person once stated, "A man convinced against his will, is of the same opinion still!"

Being a good listener is the most effective strategy in winning and maintaining acquaintances. Everyone loves a good listener. This is one of the qualities that makes Vintage People so valuable. They are good listeners, without criticizing and without arguing. People seek out good listeners who pay attention to them. Our society is crying out for good listeners who pay attention. Look at the popularity of the "psychics"! What do these people do except listen and give their clients a little personal attention? Psychologists make their livelihood by listening carefully. Much of what I do as a physician involves listening closely to what patients are telling me. A couple of generations ago we didn't need psychics and psychologists. We had grandma in our extended family who performed that function very well. And you didn't have to pay her.

In conclusion, Vintage People have learned what Robert Sherwood has said: "The happiest miser on earth is the man who saves up every friend he can make." Having friends is a powerful tool for success.

THIRTEEN

SOLITUDE

Be able to be alone. Lose not the advantage of solitude.

—Sir Thomas Browne

Several years ago I was helping care for a younger man with severe diabetes. He had developed gangrene in several of the toes on his right foot. The standard medical treatments, including antibiotics had not worked well, and the orthopedic surgeon was considering amputation of his foot. He had a wife and two school-age children. In addition, he was a railroad worker, and his livelihood depended upon his ability to walk, run, and to climb on trains. Naturally he was despondent at the possibility of losing part of his foot. But without the surgery, he ran the possibility of losing his life! What a hard decision to make.

One evening I was making rounds late at the hospital. The nurse informed me that my patient just wanted to be left alone. As we stood at the nursing station discussing the medical decisions that had to be made, the hospital chaplain on call overheard us. He was a wise Vintage Person, a retired minister, whom I had known for several years. "Your patient just needs some quiet time—some solitude," he said. Then he made a statement that I have remembered ever since. He said, "Man lives in an inner world and an outer world. They are connected, but different. Right now he has to retreat into the solitude of the inner world where there are resources to deal with his crisis!"

213

What a powerful statement! Vintage People realize that there are resources in the outer world, and resources in the inner world. The most successful people know how and when to focus on one or the other. We may be transported from the outer world into the inner world by noble means such as spiritual concerns, prayer, and meditation. Other less majestic issues such as disappointment with the material world, crisis, fear, and depression will sometimes drive us to the inner world as well. This is a place that excludes the rest of the world, where we have to deal with issues ourselves. This is a place where *we* are accountable. Others cannot help. The physical world cannot help. Christianity teaches that we are born alone into this physical world, and when we leave we will stand alone before our Judge. This is the kind of place I am talking about.

There is power is this inner place! Great resources abound here that are not available in the physical world, resources we cannot find on the internet, power that cannot be found in materialism. The power of the inner world goes deep. We humans are missing out if we don't use this power. We don't want to stay there forever, but it is a great place to visit for strength. Successful Vintage People have learned how to use the power of solitude. This ability seems to come with age and maturity. As Albert Einstein said, "Solitude is painful when one is young, but delightful when one is more mature."

Silence

Have you noticed all the young people about with earphones on? My teenagers wear them almost continually—it seems to be part of their wardrobe. Compare this to the number of older people wearing headsets on. When you ride with your teenager or other younger people in their cars, the radio is almost always on. But when you ride with older people, that is seldom the case. Same thing goes for radios, televisions and stereos in the home or the workplace. At first I wondered if this was just a generation thing. But I think not. As people mature, they begin to realize the importance of silence in their lives. I'm not sure if maturity requests silence, or if silence produces maturity, but the two seem to be companions.

Vintage People have learned the importance of quiet time in their lives. "You must spend a little time in silence each day," recommended an eighty-seven-year-old lady. "It's during those times that you really get your thoughts together."

The great writer Thomas Carlye said, "Silence is the element in which great things fashion themselves together." Indeed, it seems that during periods of little or no distraction, thoughts and new ideas do come forth. If we are watching TV, listening to tapes or to the radio, our mind is restricted to thinking about that one thing. Turn off the TV, the radio, or the tapes, and in the resulting silence, our minds can soar. We are free to think about anything!

Psychologists and religious leaders recommend periods of shutting down our senses, not only to noise but to visual input as well. During those times our brain can concentrate on what is within. Dream research shows that much of our dreaming is really the mind's way of "playing back" and organizing what has happened during the day. We also know that people become mentally ill if not allowed to dream. Silence and meditation are as important to the conscious mind as dreaming is to the subconscious mind. Science has proved that our EEG—our brain waves—change during periods of silent meditation.

I have read that the three best places to get new ideas are the three "Bs"—Bed, Bathroom, and Bus. I don't ride the bus—our small town is too rural to have a bus system—but I must admit that I often come up with great ideas while in the other two places! Why is this? I think it is because here we shut down all the other inputs that our brains deal with all day. New ideas find it hard to fashion themselves when we have a steady stream of input, with no time to reflect. Rather than having to assimilate information at a rapid pace, our minds prefer to have time to reflect, to sort, and to put together new ideas in ways that they have never been thought of before. As Adlai Stevenson says, "In quiet places, reason abounds."

Norman Vincent Peale suggests that "clearing the mind" is important to good mental health. He recommends at least fifteen minutes of uninterrupted silence in everyone's life every day. Vintage People all have their individual ways of doing just that. Most have learned this habit early in life, and have kept it into the Vintage years. It has a therapeutic value, like a good medicine. Many woman I know describe getting up early—before their husbands and children. Their excuse is to get out of the bathroom first, or to fix breakfast for the family. But most of them admit that they really enjoy the quiet time that they can have alone at the beginning of the day. Many men find this time while driving to work or while commuting.

I know that on days when I am hurrying all day long and am bombarded with questions and pleas for my time from my patients, the hospital, my nursing staff, medical students, insurance companies, Medicare representatives, and pharmaceutical salesmen, I seldom get anything done except the routine. New innovations take thought, and new ideas take a silent period to arrange and present themselves.

One warning. Silence is a little like many of the medications I prescribe. The right amount is good for us, but too much is not better. Too much medication can be toxic, and so can too much silence. If we spend all of our time in quiet reflection, nothing will get done. We will lack action. Monks are an example of too much silence. They may have profound ideas emerge from their lives of silent reflection, but if that information is not passed on—if no action is taken—nothing is accomplished.

The important message here is that most Vintage People, people who are successful and live long happy lives, have worked the right amount of quiet time into their busy daily lives. They find power in solitude and silence. They have been doing it for a long time. Daily periods of silence are an inexpensive path to good mental health that we can all work into our lives.

Pauses

I've watched a lot of individuals attack life with enthusiasm and vigor, yet some were more successful than others. One of the reasons, I feel, were the pauses in their lives—the periods of rest, reflection, and renewal. God labored for six days, and then He rested, demonstrating an inherent human need that was recognized even by the ancients. We still need to pause to assimilate where we are and where we want to be. We need to retreat to where we can study our lives. Successful Vintage People realize this principle and use it in their business lives, in their relationships and even in their spiritual lives. Yet, some of us human beings feel superior even to God in that respect. We think we can push ourselves forward without a personal retreat.

I saw an article recently describing how modern labor-saving devices actually propel us into a more hurried lifestyle. Instead of having more time, we end up with less. Perhaps we didn't like the time required to bake bread, to cook a meal without a microwave, or to write letters and wait days or weeks for a reply, but our brain enjoyed the assimilation time.

When stimuli are bombarding us from all directions, Vintage People stop, pause, and seem to take a deep breath and then look over the situation. They figure the best way to proceed, where to best focus their energy. As a medical student, I was overwhelmed by information and all the tasks to complete. Days and weeks were simply a blur. I was always behind on what I needed to learn. Everything seemed to be an emergency and needed to be done immediately. I loved the excitement of jumping into a "code blue" and doing cardiopulmonary resuscitation, starting IVs, putting in arterial lines, and all the other procedures that students learn. We felt we were really helping mankind.

As I matured in my medical education, I learned that few things in life are immediate. In the emergency room during my first year of residency, I remember busily working on a patient, as we had been trained. The attending physician came in and looked over the entire situation. He studied the laboratory work and checked the cardiac monitors. Finally, he told us to stop what we were doing. The patient was dying from a terminal illness and had requested in writing not to be resuscitated. We had been too busy doing things to check the big picture. I vividly remember the comment my attending physician made: "It's like someone just winds you interns up and you start pounding on someone's chest! For God's sake, stand back every now and then and look at what you are doing!" I've remembered those words.

As I matured in the field of medicine, I found that most illnesses and other medical problems, actually got better or went away completely if I did nothing at all. I think that is what Hippocrates meant when he warned the medical profession to, above all, "do no harm." There are only a few times when emergency efforts are truly needed. The wise physician, as well as other wise persons, will pause and assimilate what is happening around them and then act appropriately.

Vintage People don't wait for annual vacations to renew themselves. They take pauses throughout the day and throughout the week. One gentleman that I consider a true Vintage Person sums it up like this: "When you take pauses throughout the day, you will feel much more like the master of your universe and less like a controlled puppet dancing to an ever increasing pace." There is a choice!

FOURTEEN

SPIRITUALITY

"I have been driven many times to my knees by the overwhelming conviction that I had nowhere else to go."

—Abraham Lincoln

On my hospital rounds one day a few weeks ago, the nurses pointed out to me that it was one of my patient's eighty-seventh birthday. She had spent her birthday in the hospital's skilled nursing unit recovering from surgery after a fractured hip. Her spirits remained high and, according to the staff, she had experienced a wonderful birthday with a shower of cards, lots of flowers, and balloons. As I noticed her room packed with all these items of celebration, I made the comment, "It looks like turning eighty-seven hasn't bothered you a bit!"

"No," she replied. "You see, getting older is something I think I am really good at!"

Indeed, she is very good at getting older. She is a Vintage Person. As I left her room, the young medical student following me wondered out loud, "Why would anyone celebrate getting older? Aren't they just getting that much closer to death—to the end? It's weird that people want to celebrate at that age!"

My student had a lot to learn about becoming a Vintage Person, much to learn about medicine, and a lot to learn about life.

I'm involved with the medical school in what is called a "community health rotation." I don't expect students to learn a lot of the latest scientific information on this rotation. I've been out of medical school too long to be current on the latest theories, and the students seem to get plenty of that at the University of Kansas School of Medicine anyway. But I do want them to learn the "art" of medicine and people skills in healing.

Because of his attitude, I made sure this particular student spent some time during his rotation with several of my patients who were receiving hospice care. That may seem like a strange thing to do, but I've learned that terminally ill people who have accepted their mortality celebrate life to the fullest. I wanted this student to see that. He expected the hospice patients to be serious, grim and depressed. Instead, he found laughter, peace, and almost daily celebrations of the little things in life that we tend to take for granted. In the midst of suffering and facing death square in the face—even expecting death at any time—people were celebrating life.

"I was able to walk across the room today by myself," one lady with terminal cancer told him. Another patient celebrated the fact that he was able to talk on the phone for the first time since his tracheotomy. Still another man who was losing his eyesight because of an inoperable brain tumor commented, "I watched the sunset today, and will cherish its beauty always."

By the end of the one-month rotation, my student's attitude had changed. During the exit interview that I always have with my students, I asked him what was the most important thing he had learned. He answered, "Doctor Old, you have shown me that the human spirit is stronger than any disease, and I need to always recognize that fact as I treat patients!"

He got an "A!"

To really understand the importance of this characteristic—the human spirit, let's look at the history of mankind. Early on, mankind gets kicked out of the Garden of Eden. Adam and Eve receive the knowledge that they are mortal and will die. To my knowledge, human beings are the only creatures on earth that realize they will die. Later on, Galileo deflates our ego even more by telling us we are not the center of the universe. We are not even in a very good galactic neighborhood! Darwin tells us we descended from monkeys, and Freud tells us we are all crazy! Bummer! What is there to be happy about? Why would the human race want to go on? Why do we want to bring children into this world? Why do we celebrate getting older? Getting older should reasonably lead to profound depression, as my medical student first acknowledged.

Indeed, if the value of our life were measured by physical possessions, I think our species would have given up long ago. That is not enough to make us want to survive. Obviously, human existence goes beyond the physical. All physicians, if they are to be good healers, should recognize the existence of the human spirit. It is the wonderful endowment of the human spirit that finds life purposeful.

Believe in a higher power

From the very earliest human writings and the very earliest archeological findings of human history, it appears that every culture has had a belief in some kind of an afterlife. It may have taken different forms, but the basic belief was there. In our culture that belief affects human behavior in this current life, particularly as we age and become Vintage People.

The Gallup Poll, conducted by George Gallup Jr. and his colleagues, investigated the spiritual beliefs of Americans over the past sixty years. The data has been fairly steady over that period of time. According to his polls, ninety-five percent of Americans believe in God. Eighty eighty percent believe that the Bible is the actual or inspired Word of God. Seventy-two percent say that their whole approach to life is based on their spiritual and religious views. Fifty-seven percent say they pray regularly, and forty-two percent attend some type of church or other religious service regularly.

All this to say that Americans do think about and act on their religious beliefs. For Vintage People religious faith is one of their leading characteristics. Although my surveys were not as scientific as the Gallop Poll, every one of the Vintage People that I interviewed placed spirituality as a major reason for their longevity and their happiness. If we did a survey that was more scientific, perhaps the percentage would be lower, maybe ninety percent. But even then, spirituality and religion in their lives is highly significant. It is a characteristic of Vintage People that we must pay attention to and learn from.

Carl Jung, one of the founders of modern psychiatry, summarized much of his clinical work with this confession: "Among all my patients in the second half of life...there has not been one whose problem in the last resort was not that of finding a religious outlook on life...none of them has been really healed who did not regain his religious outlook."

Herbert Benson, M.D., in his research on spirituality and healing at Harvard Medical School, feels that human beings are "wired for God." He believes that somewhere in our very genes and DNA humans are programmed to have a spiritual nature, a desire to seek out a power greater than ourselves, a desire to believe in the hope of an afterlife, a desire to feel spiritual significance is programmed into our computer-like brains when we are born. We know now that our minds function somewhat like a computer, assimilating all that is around us, and then sorting and storing that information. We also know that when we are born, certain basic human characteristics, or "instincts" (a word I don't like to associate with people) are already there for survival. Sucking, eating, a fear of falling, grasping, and a desire for love are a few of these pre-programmed characteristics. Spirituality is harder to measure, but it is there and, just like the other characteristics, is good for survival. It is something that keeps human beings going in tough times. Our spiritual side adds hope and purpose to life, even though we know we are mortal. It helps us survive. How ironic that Western medicine and science have ignored the force that gives humans the desire to live!

We seek spirituality because it is good for our health and good for our life. Some say that God designed us this way. He put a yearning in our soul to seek Him. The atheist or agnostic would say that this characteristic is something that has evolved as a survival technique for humans. Either way, it is real and it is important. Vintage People have discovered this through living. It is exciting that science seems to be rediscovering the human soul as well. Experiments with prayer and healing are showing amazing positive results.

Religion

An eighty-one-year-old nurse who has traveled extensively in the Peace Corps has seen many countries and experienced many cultures, writes, "Does it matter if one is Buddhist, Hindu, or Christian? I think not, as long as one has faith. I would find it very depressing if I thought that after death there is nothing—that's all there is. We need faith. It would be difficult to go it alone."

This sums up the feelings of most Vintage People. As they mature and age, they develop an awareness of their spirituality. It would be hard to face aging alone, but most Vintage People do not feel they are doing it alone. What a tremendous coping mechanism God has given us. As they observe life and participate in life over the years, it becomes clearer to them that we are not alone in our sojourn here on this planet.

M. Scott Peck, M.D., writing in his best selling book, *The Road Less Traveled and Beyond*, states, "As a scientist, I expect statistical proof whenever possible to convince me of most things. But as I continue to mature, I've become more and more impressed by the frequency of statistically highly improbable events. In their very improbability, I began to see the fingerprints of God."

One of my Vintage Patients described it this way; "As I age, I'm not sure there are accidents!"

Spirituality is the huge umbrella under which such things as religion are covered. There is one human spirituality, but many religions. Religion differs from spirituality in that religion has rules. It is an organized part of spirituality. Religion offers explanations of the unseen and is a guide of life. Religion is a specific way that people see spirituality.

The word "spirituality" comes from the Latin *spirare,* "to breathe." It involves mystical insights of the human mind with nature, with other people, and with a Supreme Being or Power. Such things as faith, hope, love, courage, trust, and peace are included under this broad topic. Religion is a way to nurture spirituality. Religion involves community, whereas spirituality is more individual and less structured. Most religions contain a system of beliefs, symbols, and practices that help connect us with ourselves, with other people, and with the deity.

As Vintage People describe their spirituality, it seems to encompass more than even this broad definition of religion. For some, spirituality involves a sense of awe and mystery. One Vintage Person I know well is a Native American. He describes the following as a very spiritual experience: "Spirituality can be felt on a quiet spring morning standing alone in an open field, watching the sunrise, hearing the wind, seeing the clouds and hills in the distance, listening to the birds and other animals, and just knowing I am part of the earth."

If you haven't tried that, you should. Take it from a farm boy, it is a very spiritual experience.

To me, planting a garden is spiritual. Watching the miracle of a birth is spiritual. I can make an incision in the human body, and it heals. I don't know how it heals, but the cells have a DNA blueprint for healing—that is spiritual to me. Gazing into the night sky is a spiritual experience. Who could lie gazing into the night sky with all the billions of stars and not feel a since of spirituality, a sense of awe, a sense of mystery?

Studying the human body is a spiritual experience. I guess you would know what I mean if you had dissected a cadaver like I have. I know what muscle tissue looks like. I know what an artery looks like. I know what nerve tissue looks like. I've seen human intestines, gall bladders, kidneys and other internal organs. I've seen a beating human heart—something most have not seen. When we removed a patient's cranium in neurosurgery, and I was privileged to gaze down at the gray-white convolutions of the human brain, I knew right there that God had planted a mind—a

human spirit—probably the most powerful force in this
universe. That, to me, was a spiritual experience.

God's handiwork is obvious in humans. I'm convinced
that the human body and mind could no more happen by
accident or evolve without some special guiding force than
one could pile a mass of plastic, metal, and electric wires
into a junk yard, and have them fall together in such a way
as to create a computer or the space shuttle. There is too
much detail in the human body. Look at eyelashes. They
help keep bits of dust and other foreign matter out of our
eyes. I doubt that our species would have come to a
screeching halt in evolution if we did not have them. Fin-
gernails are a great asset, but hardly have survival implica-
tions. Likewise, our nasal passages warm the air we
breathe, sweat glands cool us, shivering warms us, vocal
cords serve not only a function for communication but can
also be trained to perform beautiful music simply for pleasure. All of these things seem to be accessories beyond
what the basic human body needed purely for survival of
the species.

As a physician, I see both medicine and spirituality as
dealing with the reality of human fragility. Religious traditions provide us with belief systems and coping skills to
survive this fragility. After all, we are in a hostile world,
medically speaking. Every day, billions of bacteria attack
us. Were it not for the continual battle of our immune system, we could not survive.

Illness reminds us of how vulnerable we really are.
Immanuel Jakobovits, Chief Rabbi of the British Common-
wealth of Nations, in his classic work, *Jewish Medical Eth-
ics,* writes that "disease forges an especially close link
between God and man; the Divine Presence Itself, as it
were, rests on the head of the sickbed!"

Theologians explain this fact by saying that people try to protect themselves through religion which provides order and control over our lives. We have no ultimate control over sickness. Therefore, many sick or hurting patients call out to some higher being in the universe who, they hope, does have things under control. This human vulnerability forces us into our spiritual side. Said another way, "There are no atheists in foxholes!"

For the same reason, perhaps, we can also say there are few atheists in old age. The Vintage People I have interviewed are convinced that religion is good for them and for all of us. It is good for our mental health, it is good for our physical health, it is good for one's marriage, it is even good for our day-to-day living with other people.

Most religious traditions provide coping skills. They encourage good health habits, a wholesome life-style, and a supportive community. I find it fascinating to read the health laws in the Old Testament. It is a miracle that they could have been written three thousand years ago. As a modern physician, I am amazed by how healthful these rules were. The people living then had no idea of sanitation, the germ theory, or the health risks of abusive living. Yet their health laws were scientifically correct. Most of the foods that were considered unclean, really were unclean at that time. Pork was especially dangerous at that time. Predatory birds were likely disease carriers. Even today, shellfish remain carriers of hepatitis, and frequent causes of food poisoning and enteritis. These foods were all prohibited. What about ritual handwashing? It's no longer a ritual, but we realize the great health benefits of it. Personal hygiene and even quarantine regulations are described in these Judeo-Christian scriptures, long before it was known that diseases were contagious.

The advice about human relations in the Bible is no less miraculous. Modern psychologists are just rediscovering how these laws work. Forgiveness is good for you. Being faithful to your spouse is good for you. Prayer, faith, and the support of church members are good for you. Hope in the future is good for you. Serving others is good for you. If you think for a moment of the influential Vintage People that you know—those Vintage People who serve as a light in someone's life—most all of them are religious. They may not all attend organized religious services regularly, but even those who don't still consider themselves "religious."

Spiritual beliefs and religion make life better. And it is a win-win situation. If there is no God or afterlife, so what? By practicing religion, you have made this life better. But if there is a loving Creator in the universe, then we have even more to look forward to. Vintage People have discovered that they win either way.

Science and spirituality

Dr. Norman Vincent Peale said, "Religious faith may very well be considered a science, for it responds invariably to certain formulae. Perform the technique of faith according to the laws which have been proved workable in human experience and you will always get a result of power."

Science is beginning to rediscover the human spirit or soul. I recently attended a conference sponsored by Harvard Medical School on the spiritual aspects of healing. Such a conference for doctors would have been unheard of when I was doing my medical training about twenty years ago. An amazing amount of scientific information was presented about the effects of prayer and the importance of the human spirit in healing. Most major religions were represented at the meeting and are represented in ongoing research that is being done.

Let me digress a minute and explain what has happen in the field of medicine, because it parallels society's thinking about spirituality and the human body. Until the seventeenth century, the field of medicine pretty much accepted the fact that the mind and the body were one. Treatments often relied on the beliefs of the patient and the placebo effect. Many cures worked, as long as the doctor and patient believed they would work. All kinds of things were tried. It is fun, yet a little scary, to read medical history.

We laugh now at bleeding, leaches, and purging. But these procedures are credited with healing thousands of people. Even the moss that grew on the skulls of hanged prisoners in England brought a premium price at one time and was used to cure such things as tuberculosis. It would be interesting to see what is written about our modern medicine in another hundred years!

In the seventeenth century the French philosopher René Descartes suggested that the body did not need the mind to function. He felt the body was a machine-like organism of chemical reactions and that its functioning could be explained totally on a scientific basis. As modern techniques, medications, and surgery progressed, it did seem that the human body was a machine with replaceable parts. Many of our therapies began to work on the body without the beliefs of a person's mind. General anesthesia worked, no matter what a patient's belief system was. Penicillin worked, pacemakers worked, hip replacements worked, and the human spirit was forgotten. I was taught in medical school that patient's beliefs and spirituality just got in the way when scientific doctors were trying to do their jobs. Prayer was okay, so long as it didn't delay what we as doctors knew was best for the patient.

In the eighteenth century, a diagnosis of pneumonia in someone over fifty years of age was worse than a diagnosis of cancer is today. It was a death warrant. Prayer was the only treatment. Suddenly, with one shot of penicillin, these people could be cured. This discovery was not that long ago. As a young physician I remember talking to older physicians who lived at the time when antibiotic use became widespread. They reported that pneumonia victims who were in respiratory distress and moribund, near death, were given this wonder drug. Not only were they better by the next day, but many patients who had been given up for dead the night before were up walking the halls the next morning! These were truly miracles.

Penicillin was in such demand and was so expensive that the urine of patients given the drug was saved and the penicillin extracted from it to give to other patients. And it worked—even after passing through several patients!

Likewise, general anesthesia and modern surgery was born. The miracles continued! And society loved it. The patient's belief system and spirituality were ignored. It didn't matter what you believed or didn't believe; these miracles of medicine worked. If you were given a general anesthetic, you went to sleep—no question about it.

From this technology of wonders, one thing did get lost—the patient's spirituality and belief systems. Fortunately, we are now rediscovering the importance of these factors as they affect healing and treating the whole person—mind, body, and soul. Society is beginning to rediscover the importance of the human spirit. It's not that we don't appreciate the miracles of modern medicine, but now that the newness of the miracles is wearing off, we are asking, "Isn't there more to human beings than the body?" It is ironic that science, the very culprit that drew our attention away from the spirit and onto the physical body, is now pushing us back toward rediscovering the soul. Scientific study is leading us back toward religion. Religion has not led us back toward science.

Science is showing that a patient's belief system and spiritual nature are important in healing. We are again trying to tap that power to help with healing. Notice I said "to help with healing." I don't think we should throw away the miracles of medicine. Why not use both? It is reported that at one time the prophet Muhammadan was asked if people should seek healing through spiritual means or through medicines. He said, "Yes, you must seek remedy from medicine, because whatever disease God has created in this world, He has also created its remedy as well."

One of the landmark research projects that has started to pull science back toward spirituality was published in the *Southern Medical Journal* in 1988 by Randolf Byrd. He essentially divided patients in the hospital coronary care unit into two groups. Neither the patients nor the staff knew which were in which groups. He then had a group of people meet and pray for one group of patients. The patients didn't know they were being prayed for. The results, when tabulated, were so astonishing that they were published. What Dr. Byrd found was that in 393 patients, the group that was prayed for had far fewer complications and left the hospital earlier. No patient in the prayed-for group ended up on a respirator, while twelve patients in the other group did. The group that was prayed for also had less pneumonia and required fewer medications and antibiotics. Something was clearly going on here! Now there are numerous scientific studies that are confirming the same results.

While some might think that it is "not right" to try to prove that prayer works, or that spirituality really does help with healing, science marches on. Society is moving along with this. The interest in "near death" experiences and in angels has peaked over the last few years. Granted, many of us know prayer and spirituality are real without having to prove it, but what does it matter if people arrive at this conclusion by different means? I may see a mountain in the distance and know there is snow on top, while someone else may have to climb that mountain and actually touch the snow to believe it. But we both reach the correct assumption that there is snow on the mountain.

Research on the healing effects of prayer has created a bit of a dilemma for physicians. If we know that religion or other aspects of spirituality are good for a patient's health, how do we approach that very personal topic? I don't feel that spirituality and religion should be imposed upon the patient, but neither should we reduce the person affected by illness to a purely biologic entity. Freedom is essential for meaningful spirituality. It cannot be forced upon someone. I've heard religion described as being like a toothbrush— everyone needs one, but everyone should have his own!

If physicians impose their own religious views or pray for patients in one way or another, Larry Dossey, M.D., and author of *Prayer is Good Medicine,* says, "Quite simply, it is a shameful abuse of power." Dossey suggests reliance on the clergy—or referral to them—something we physicians are good at doing.

Spirituality and health are connected in various ways that are still being scientifically clarified, but spirituality does have the power to change our health and how we enjoy this thing we call life. Even the most saintly people are fragile—they get sick. The greatest guru dies.

When I was a third year medical student, this message really came home to me. The medical center was rolling out the red carpet for a renowned state senator, who also was on the board of regents of the medical school. I was assigned to take care of him! As a student, it was my job to do the admitting history and complete physical exam. I was nervous when I first met this distinguished gentleman, but once I started the physical exam, and he had his clothes off, I began to see him as just another human being. He expressed the same concerns about his health that we all have. I realized how important our health is to us when he began telling me about his difficulty with his prostate and his difficulty urinating. It seemed bizarre to be talking to such an important and distinguished man about something as earthy as urination and the size of his prostate! I realized that we are all in this life together, and no matter how powerful or famous we become, we are still limited by our human fragility.

As science has started to explore the relationships between our physical bodies and our spiritual side, several important facts have emerged. First of all, there is overwhelming evidence that there is more to a human being than just his physical presence. Whether this mysterious power or energy is assigned to spirituality, to God, to the power of the universe, or to purely unknown physical principles, it is obvious that something is involved with human satisfaction, with healing, and with life, that we do not yet understand.

Science is proving that religion makes life better. But it is also showing that no specific religion owns spirituality. Science is discovering that *all* religions seem to function equally well when it comes to such things as healing and satisfaction of life.

When the effects of prayer are studied, as mentioned above, prayer makes a positive difference in peoples lives. However, it is interesting that when the people doing the praying are evaluated, it does not seem to make any difference if they are Baptist, Catholic, Jewish, Islamic, Hindu, Buddhist or are members of any other organized religion.

These studies have been repeated many times, and there is no doubt that people of different faiths can get equally good results from prayer. What does seem to matter is the belief or commitment of the person doing the praying. Those that believe in what they are doing have the best results! From a Christian perspective, I don't find that surprising. Jesus understood that principle well and taught it to His followers. In Matthew 21:22, He says, "And all things, whatsoever ye shall ask in prayer, believing, ye shall receive." And when other religions are studied, this is one of the prevailing themes. If you are committed and believe in what you are doing, it works.

Prayer

Research by the Gallop Poll shows that meditative prayer increases with age. Forty-five percent of persons aged 18 to 24 pray regularly, while seventy percent of 65-year-olds do so. More women than men report praying regularly, and more Afro-Americans pray regularly than whites.

In keeping with these statistics, then, one would expect to find the most information on prayer from older, black, females. In my interviews that was the case. People in these categories seemed to answer questions in a more spiritual way than other people did. Because I live in a predominantly Christian culture, people I know best approach prayer from the Christian perspective, but I recognize that prayer is by no means limited to this perspective.

In summary, almost Vintage People who pray all had specific times of the day to pray—the most common time was before bed. They also prayed through the day whenever the need arose. They felt that God was close to them, not far off. They were not afraid to ask for specific things when they prayed, but also very often just gave thanks and said, "Thank you, Lord," or "Praise the Lord!"

They generally prayed in their own language and did not feel it was important to use any kind of formal words. There was some ritual involved, but most said they just "talked to God" as a friend, without going though a lot of preparatory ritual. Hymns, however, were important and were commonly used as praise or to prepare for prayer.

Everyone agreed that negative prayers don't work. Prayers had to be positive and in accordance with the will of God. They could recite numerous prayers that had been answered and had no question that their prayers were heard. But they agreed that they were always prepared to "take whatever the good Lord gives me."

One lady gave me an excellent statement as to what prayer is not. "Prayer is not," she said, "going to a church building, where I kneel and close my eyes, to talk to some far off, white, male, judgmental, parent figure, who prefers to be addressed in English!"

No indeed! According to the Vintage People I asked, prayer can be done anywhere, anytime, under any circumstances, and by anyone. They also see God as a personal friend who is always near and always ready to hear from his "children." There is no monopoly on prayer. And Vintage People agree that prayer is good for them, as well as for the people they pray for. It helps physically and mentally, as well as spiritually.

In his *Essays on Faith and Morals,* William James said, "The exercise of prayer, in those who habitually exert it, must be regarded by doctors as the most adequate and normal of all the pacifiers of the mind and calmers of the nerves." Science is now proving that this is true.

Science has a hard time getting a handle on why prayer doesn't work all the time. When an apple drops from a tree, it always falls down at a predictable rate. Objects in space are predictable in their orbits. A chemical reaction happens the same way every time. It has to be this way in the physical universe or everything would collapse or become chaotic.

Why is it, then, that prayers sometimes work, and sometimes they don't? I have seen a hospital room filled with relatives praying for a loved one around the clock. Their faith was so great that they even refused to believe that the patient was dead, although it was a physical reality. They had no lack of faith, yet their loved one did indeed die! The most saintly people have hardships and die.

Some of our prayers, because of our shortsightedness are not really in our best interests. Some may even be detrimental to us or to other people, or to God's will. Some prayers are impossible for God to grant. I always use the example of my praying for the Kansas Jayhawk basketball team to win when there are just as many fans on the other side praying for Kansas State to win! What's God to do in that situation?

Some of our prayers would do us in if they were granted. C.S. Lewis writes, "If God had granted all the silly prayers I've made in my life, where should I be now?" Think about that! If every prayer was immediately answered in the affirmative, what would you be? You certainly would not be human. If all my prayers had been answered, there would have been a pony in my living room under the Christmas tree on Christmas morning, when I was eight years old!

Vintage People have come to accept that it would not be good for us to get everything we ever wanted. But that does not mean prayer is ineffective or that prayer does not have some real, scientific basis. One retired aviator explained his version of this concept to me as follows: "The weather also conforms to scientific laws. Yet it is extremely hard to accurately predict. I think prayer is a lot like that. There are just too many things going on that we don't understand, but that doesn't mean that there are not laws of the universe involved."

I suppose it is like the placebo effect. Sometimes the effects are significant, but not always. Sometimes it rains when it is predicted, but sometimes it doesn't—at least in Kansas! In the spiritual realm, there are so many variables at play that the outcomes are sometimes hard for us to understand. Vintage People learn to accept this. They don't give up on their spirituality just because certain things happen or don't happen. They sense there is great power in prayer, a power that we as humans are just beginning to realize. They also realize that we will never understand all the mystery involved in our lifetimes.

As Paul wrote to the Corinthians two thousand years ago, "For now we see in a mirror dimly, but then face to face. Now I know in part; then I shall understand fully, even as I have been fully understood."

FIFTEEN

GOING HOME

"For everything there is a season...a time to be
born,
and a time to die."
—Ecclesiastes 3:1-2

D eath was the subject that I was most hesitant to ask
Vintage People about. My fears were unfounded. My subjects were willing to share their thoughts on death with me.
Vintage People have reached a remarkable acceptance of
death. They do not ignore death nor do they become
obsessed with it. Each has reached a personal conclusion
about death, and they all feel that they understand it. They
realize that death is one of the things in life that they cannot
change. They therefore accept it. As one of my Vintage
Patients put it, "I'm not afraid of dying, but I'm not in a
hurry either!"

As mentioned in the last chapter, humans are the only
species on this planet that realize we are going to die. What
an awesome responsibility to deal with. I've found that different people handle this knowledge of mortality in different
ways. Children, for example, see death as something so
remote that they don't have to think about it. But when
death does strike close to children, they are usually very
accepting—much like Vintage People. Teens usually see
themselves as invincible and therefore ignore death. When
I've tried to talk with young adults about death, I've noticed
that they push away and change the subject. They are

uncomfortable and often tell me, "I don't want to talk about this." They even hesitate to use the word.

But whenever I have had to approach the subject of death with Vintage People, I find that they have thought about death. As a matter of fact, through their maturity and participating in the "art of living," they have figured out death to their own satisfaction. They have a concept of what is going to happen to them as well as to their loved ones. This is probably because no one reaches Vintage status without coming close to death—the death of parents, friends, loved ones, spouses, and acquaintances. Most have had situations in their own lives where they felt their own mortality—the "close calls" of life. They have been forced to think about death.

Medically speaking

There is an old adage in medicine: "All bleeding stops—eventually!" I guess that is a little bit like dying. Everyone accepts death—eventually!

Several recent surveys asked Americans what they hoped they would die from. Almost all listed a quick death. The overwhelming majority hoped to die painlessly in their sleep. If that couldn't happen, then they hoped it would be a heart attack—something fast. I had one of my professors in medical school tell our class, "I used to worry that I might die of a heart attack. As I've gotten older, I now worry that I won't!" In studying the history of medicine, I was surprised to find that prior to this century, sudden death was what people feared most. All through history, people have hoped for the chance to be prepared for their death—to have a chance to take care of those last-minute details. They wanted a chance to have their families around, and to say good-bye. Perhaps the medical profession is to blame for this change of attitude toward the process of dying. I am afraid that sometimes we prolong dying rather than extending life. In medical school we learned the universal stages of a dying patient, as first observed by Dr. Elizabeth Kubler-Ross. All patients seem to follow this pattern if they have time in the dying process. These stages include, first of all, denial. Anger, bargaining, and depression follow. But the most encouraging thing to me is that the final step is acceptance. The patient seems at last to bow to his sentence and following that enters a peaceful, calm and beautiful time.

I have seen this so many times in dealing with dying patients in my practice. The first response is usually, "No, not me. I can beat this!" During this time patients may get other doctors' opinions and search for a cure. They may try chemotherapy, surgery, radiation, or less conventional therapies. I've had patients travel to other countries seeking cures where they are taken advantage of by quackery.

Once they find that nothing is going to work, that the diagnosis is right, and that their time on earth is limited, most patients then get angry. "Why me? Why not somebody else? I've got too much to live for!" These patients are often obnoxious and hard to care for. Even their families sometimes have trouble being sympathetic.

When a difficult patient suddenly becomes cooperative, it signals the next stage, which is bargaining. After the denial, and after the anger, the patient finally decides that if they do everything they are told, maybe they can get a cure. They suddenly do everything the doctor tells them. During this time they usually bargain with God to have one more chance to do something important, one more day without pain, or one more chance of a cure. During this stage, I've seen one patient schedule appointments with a priest, a rabbi, and a Baptist minister—all in one day.

If bargaining does not work, the patient sinks into a depression. This is a normal grief reaction to the losses they are about to experience. After all, they are about to lose their own body image and everyone they love. There may be financial burdens and a tremendous feeling of needing to get everything in order. This is the stage where suicide is often contemplated or carried out.

Finally the time for acceptance arrives. This is the stage I want to emphasize. Vintage People seem to reach this stage rapidly. They can sometimes even skip some of the stages above and arrive at acceptance unscathed by the other stages. Vintage People, I think, have already worked through these other stages long ago. They have already arrived at acceptance—the final stage. When I asked a group of Vintage People what their reaction would be if I told them they would die soon, one woman responded, "Hallelujah, I'm going home!" Another shouted out, "I'm ready!" And another even replied, "I don't know what has taken so long!"

I have been privileged to be present when people die. In previous generations that would not be a unique privilege. People previously died at home, surrounded by their loved ones, and families got to experience death. But in our culture, most people die in institutions, often with only the medical profession around. Therefore, I feel it is a privilege to witness death, just as I feel it is a privilege to be present for the birth of a baby. Sharing these special times is one of the great benefits of being a family physician that goes far beyond any financial or physical rewards.

I have been at the bedside of more people at the actual time of death than most people. What I have observed gives me great confidence as I think about my own death. I think Vintage People understand this. The deaths I have witnessed have been peaceful when death finally comes.

Prior to the end, there may be pain and distress, but when death is actually near—when it is inevitable, there is a great peace that comes over patients. Every patient that I have been with at the time of death reached this level of peaceful acceptance if given time. Of course, patients brought to the emergency room suffering from a gunshot wound or other major trauma where death is almost instantaneous don't have time to reach this level. But if it is allowed, the natural course of dying includes a peaceful ending.

The timing of death may not be totally random. As a physician I have often seen people die soon after some significant event they had been "living for." I remember a patient who defied all odds, staying alive until her youngest daughter arrived at the bedside—and died just as she heard her daughter's voice. History tells us that both Plato and Buddha died on their birthdays. More recently, American forefathers Thomas Jefferson and John Adams both died on the Fourth of July—the fiftieth anniversary of the signing of the Declaration of Independence. Jefferson's last words were, "This is the Fourth?"

In contrast, I have experienced the death of patients who were not expected to die. Their medical conditions could not totally explain their death. Some simply "gave up." I have learned that if a patient tells me they are going to die, they are probably right. A Vintage Nun told me, "The soul decides when it is time to go. And when it is time, it will find a way out, even if it has to use cancer, an accident, or failure of the immune system!"

Whatever the cause, at the time of death patients often look peaceful, smile, and make statements such as, "I see Jesus now!" I remember one dying lady who had been widowed several years earlier smiling and saying, "Oh, there is Henry coming to greet me!" Another began naming family members who had died earlier; according to the family, these names were accurate.

I recall vividly a Vintage Gentleman I cared for early in my medical career. He was six foot three inches tall, and had been a star basketball player for the University of Kansas. At the time he played he was the tallest player on the team—which shows how long ago that was. I always enjoyed talking with him and had cared for him as a physician and friend for years. Now he had been in a coma for about a week, dying from kidney failure. It was his wish that we not try heroics and let him die peacefully. He had not responded to anyone for at least a week. I went into his room one morning on rounds, and talked to him for a few minutes, as was my custom. To my amazement, he opened his eyes and said, "Well, hello, Doc!" The nurse and I were dumbfounded. A second or two passed, and he looked at me again and said: "I want you to know that I'm okay!" He then just seemed to fade back and the color literally drained from his face. We stood there waiting for him to take another breath—but he did not. I remember this very well because his blood urea nitrogen was around 200. Normally, patients are in total coma when this poison builds to over 100 in their bodies. Medically and scientifically, it was impossible for him to come out of the coma and speak that clearly to us. But he did!

Such events have prejudiced me. I know science tries to explain such things as hallucinations of an oxygen-deprived brain, or just a phenomenon of dying. But after being with so many people who say similar things at the time of death, I am convinced that they indeed do see something that I cannot see. I am convinced that what they see is a pleasant thing. Henry Wadsworth Longfellow stated it beautifully when he wrote, "…and as the evening twilight fades away, the sky is filled with stars invisible by day."

Science has difficulty accepting the things it cannot explain or understand. But science is not inconsistent with what I am observing in dying patients. The challenge is scientifically to verify what spirituality and religion already know. Otherwise, as physicians, we may expose our patients to misbeliefs and quackery. After all, there are lots of things that we don't understand, and we must guard against being closed minded.

Raymond A. Moody, Jr., M.D., an American psychiatrist, researched what has been described as "near death" experiences. This phenomenon has made its way into everyday American thinking. I have seen people with near death experiences twice in my career. One night in a busy emergency room where I was a resident, I helped take care of a middle-aged lady who had been in a horrible auto accident. She was "Code Blue" when she arrived, and I didn't expect her to live. She did respond to therapy in the emergency room, and we later got her stabilized enough to go to surgery. About a week later I changed services and was assigned to the orthopedic ward where this lady was recovering. I walked into her room and introduced myself. Her response surprised me. "Oh, yes," she said, "I remember you. You helped work on me when they brought me in. I read your name tag, and thought that 'Dr. Old' was a really funny name for such a young doctor!"

I was surprised that she could remember anything about her stay in the ER and asked her about it. She said, "I haven't told anyone this, and probably shouldn't tell you, because you will think I am crazy. But while you were working on me the other night, I was watching from above. I even remember what you were saying."

She then recited conversations and events in the emergency room with astonishing accuracy. I encouraged her to tell me more, and she was able even to describe the ambulance drivers who picked her up. She continued, "After the accident, I remember looking down at my smashed car, and hearing sirens coming. I was just kind of floating there and wasn't really aware of time. I was very comfortable, but a little scared. I followed the ambulance to the hospital, floating above it. I remember the big number '17' on top—for the police helicopters to identify it, I guess. Then in the emergency room I remember you!"

After I left her room, I couldn't wait to run to the Emergency Room and check the records. She was indeed brought in by ambulance "17." And when I checked to see which paramedic crew was working that night, my patient had described them exactly. Needless to say, that made quite an impression on a young doctor. But true to my scientific training, I didn't tell anyone about this occurrence for a number of years.

No matter what your religious beliefs or scientific bias, something happens to people when they are near death. It is a fact. And it is very real to the people it happens to. It is not like a dream. It is so real that people who have experienced it have totally changed lives from that point on—forever. No dream can be that powerful. The way we attempt to explain these "near death" experiences remains controversial. I don't see why we have to explain it at all. Whatever the reasons, once we reach a certain point in the dying process, it is peaceful and comfortable. That is the main thing that I want to know. That fact is comforting, and it gives me hope. For whatever reason, Vintage People have developed a belief system that allows them to see death without fear and with hope.

In the first century B.C., Publius wrote, "The fear of death is more to be dreaded than death itself." Vintage People have eliminated that fear, and are therefore free to enjoy the time they have on this planet to the fullest extent. That is their goal. If their beliefs allow freedom to enjoy living, then what difference does it make if it can be explained scientifically?

The American way

English is the only major language in the world where the word "death" means extinction or a permanent end. In most other languages the word used for death refers to a transition, a merging, or a transporting from one place to another. This reflects how Americans deal with death.

Currently, eighty percent of the people in this country die in hospitals. The American way to die is in a sterile institution. Dying is often hidden and not seen as a spiritual event. Even health care professionals are often uncomfortable talking about death. Our society seems to confirm what Henry Fielding wrote in 1751 when he said, "It hath been often said, that it is not death, but dying which is terrible."

An eighty-six-year-old patient of mine was in the hospital dying of prostate cancer. His young Methodist minister—age twenty-seven—came to call on him. My patient had a number of questions about dying and thought that he had found someone to talk to. But every time he brought up the topic, the minister changed the subject by saying things like: "You are going to be fine," and, "Don't give up!"

"I knew I was not going to be fine," the patient exclaimed later. "I knew I was going to die soon, and I wanted someone to talk to me about it!"

Finally, my patient told the minister straight forward that he would like to discuss death. At that point, the minister suggested that they pray together. As they began, my patient closed his eyes, bowed his head and prayed: "God, please help this pastor be not so afraid of death!"

This story was related to me by the minister, who told me that this experience was one of the turning points in his own life. From that point on, he studied and prayed, becoming more comfortable dealing with death. He is now a hospice chaplain and shares with dying patients on a daily basis.

In our culture, a medical and scientific environment has taken over what was previously a spiritual event. Sometimes the adoration of medical technology approaches the worship of idols. At the very least a dying patient in the hospital is likely to have IV fluids running, an oxygen mask on, a urinary catheter, and seven to ten medications being given. We still won't let the patient die unless they themselves or their families have expressly signed the appropriate "No Code Blue" documents. Patients almost have to fight to die. And once they are placed on life support, it becomes even harder.

Since CPR was discovered in the 1950s, it is considered an inherent "right" of everyone to be resuscitated if the heart stops beating. It is assumed by society that everyone wants to do everything possible to cling to life, no matter how painful or degrading that treatment may be or how poor the quality of life may be.

When a patient is admitted to a hospital, there has to be an order, signed by the doctor, for everything that is done for them. The nursing staff won't even give a Tylenol tablet or feed a patient without a specific doctor's order. I'm often called in the middle of the night for a laxative or sleeping pill. No surgical procedure, however minor, will be done without a written consent form signed by the patient and another witness.

But what about CPR? If a patient arrests, or stops breathing, we don't need a doctor's order or the patient's consent. We can give mouth-to-mouth resuscitation; stick endotracheal tubes down their throat; pound on their chest; use electrical shock treatments; put all kinds of tubes in body orifices; give all types of dangerous drugs; and even put the patient on a breathing machine. All of this is done by default—without a physician order or signed consent. The law in Kansas as well as in most states requires that life-sustaining treatment be given to anyone who does not have an advance directive should they become terminally ill and unable to communicate their wishes. Doesn't that seem backwards? If we as patients don't want all that done, then we have to have a signed order, or consent NOT to do it.

I know that CPR has saved lives and that some people recover completely after being resuscitated. Still, doing CPR to everyone unless they specifically refuse it is not good patient care. There is no other medical therapy that we perform on everybody regardless of their specific disease, age, and general medical condition. It's a little like taking out the appendix of every patient who has abdominal pain. It is great for one specific diagnosis, but won't help those patients with gall bladder disease or ulcers! CPR seems to be universal whether you have terminal cancer, heart disease, or a stroke. It's the treatment of choice if you are a marathon runner or have been in a nursing home at bed rest for twenty years. CPR is automatically triggered whether you are a newborn or are ninety-nine years old.

The way I see it, if you need CPR, you are very sick! There is no such thing as doing CPR on "healthy" people. If a patient needs resuscitation, it means they are dying, or technically have died. That implies that something is wrong! It is not just a little glitch that we can fix and then the patient can lead a normal healthy life for years to come. In reviewing the medical literature, I learned that no more than seventeen percent of patients requiring CPR in the hospital survived six months outside of a nursing home or hospital. Five to ten percent survival is more common in most hospitals.

It's exciting to watch CPR on television. It was exciting for me as a young medical student and resident. I loved to be in charge of the "paddles" and to watch the patients muscles contract as he or she heaved up on the table as we shocked them. It is indeed dramatic! But as I got a little more mature, I began to realize that someday that body on the ER cart might be me! Ask most doctors and nurses who work in the emergency room and they will tell you they want "No Code Blue" tattooed on their chests. If I have something wrong with me that is so serious that I stop breathing and my heart stops—I'm satisfied that that's the end. The treatment may be worse than the disease.

So much for my soapbox opinion. Visiting with my patients who are Vintage People, I have found that most feel this way, too. Most Vintage People that I admit to the hospital want "Do Not Resuscitate" written on their charts. As a physician, I always have to ask. This information is rarely volunteered, and most physicians don't ask. It is a hard thing to do. When I first began to approach this subject with my patients, I was fearful what they would think. Was I implying that they were so sick that they were going to die soon? After all, if your physician asks you whether or not you want resuscitation, or which funeral home you want to use, you may wonder what he or she knows! I have found that most patients do not interpret it that way at all and are often relieved that you asked. A frank discussion of their medical condition often follows, which makes us both feel better. My advice to patients is—ask your doctor about resuscitation. You will quickly learn what his or her comfort level is with this subject!

Outside the hospital the situation is even more complicated. If you have a medical emergency and dial 911, you have just ordered a whole menu of services. Some of these you may not want, and most people are unaware of them. I've seen something like the following scenario happen over and over in our community. An elderly patient slumps over or is discovered by his or her family to be unresponsive. Often the person has been sick for a couple of days, but has refused to go to the doctor. Of course, to become this ill—to be unresponsive—there has to be a severe underlying disease. Relatives don't know what to do when this happens and are frightened. They call 911!

The paramedics arrive with red lights and wailing sirens, assess the situation and begin CPR. IVs are started and drugs are given. An endotracheal tube is often placed in the sick person's throat, and artificial respirations are initiated. The paramedics start pumping on the patient's chest.

At this point, the family is scared. They don't like seeing all of this happening. After all, this is mother, or father, or grandmother, or aunt Sally, or cousin Bill. But they are too upset to do anything. Everything is progressing too fast, and the paramedics are intent upon their protocol (which is designed to fit all patients). The patient is finally transported to the hospital and placed in the intensive care unit on life support. After about three or four days of testing and evaluation, the medical staff determines that the patient has no brain activity. Now the family has to decide whether or not to "pull the plug" and disconnect their loved one from life support. Often, that decision takes a long time. If everyone is lucky, the patient may die in spite of the life support and make the decision for them. If not, this may go on for quite some time. There is a huge hospital bill, and the lives of all friends and relatives are disrupted for a long time. Death has not been prevented but prolonged.

In most states, once you call 911, you cannot tell the paramedics to stop. They won't. And they are backed by the law. The only way to prevent resuscitation is to have something in writing from a doctor *before* the 911 call is made. This written notice, at least in Kansas, has to be prominently displayed on the door of the house. It is hard to prevent someone from getting CPR and ending up on life support after that 911 call is made.

If we look at other cultures, or our own culture before the 1940s, CPR was not available, and people generally died at home. Pneumonia was called the "dying man's friend." Dehydration was welcomed. Either of these two conditions meant a painless death. When we got too ill to eat or drink, we slowly and comfortably drifted off into a coma, and died without pain.

A ninety-six year-old Vintage Gentleman was admitted to my service with a hip fracture. A few days later he developed pneumonia, a common complication. I was in the room when the nurse came in to hang his first vial of IV antibiotics. "What's that?" he asked.

"That's an antibiotic to treat your pneumonia," I replied.

"I thought pneumonia was the old man's friend," he said gruffly. "You want to take away my last friend? All the others are dead, too!" That was a wise man.

What would we have done if he had not refused? We would have treated the pneumonia so that the underlying disease could have been felt to its fullest extent. We often put IVs into people to hydrate them so they can feel every last bit of pain. I have heard other physicians tell a patient's family that they recommend an IV for comfort. What a fallacy! I've never had someone come to my office and say, "Doc, I've had a hard day. Would you please put an IV in so that I can be more comfortable!" Believe me. I've had one, and IVs are not comfortable!

Thanks to the hospice movement in this country, physicians are learning how to control pain in dying patients. We recognize that we are not going to make "junkies" out of dying patients. Science has shown that if a person is in pain and needs pain medication, they don't become addicted. Their body uses up the pain medications. Occasionally, I've had a patient on large doses of morphine or Demerol, and the chemo-therapy or radiation works. The cancer or other cause of the patient's pain goes away. I once worried that now these people who were cured from their disease would be addicted to my medications. They are not! Once the pain is gone, they don't want the medication anymore. They have no withdrawal symptoms. Compassion seems to be the best course of action. I love the creed of the old family doctor: "The physician's job is to heal sometimes; to comfort often; and to care always." This saying has never gone out of style.

Vintage people see death as positive

"We are spending our children's inheritance," is the popular bumper sticker I see on RVs, vans, and motor homes, while traveling the interstate. This is a somewhat humorous approach that some Vintage People have taken to the inevitable fact of mortality. That is one way of estate planning.

I am not surprised to find that Vintage People plan well and that most have made out a will sometime in their lives. This comes under the category of planning for the future, which we have discussed. I did not expect to find that Vintage People are often creative in their wills. Rather than being conservative and just leaving all their possessions to children or relatives, they tend to do things that enhance their lives while they are still living, things that they can be proud of now. This gives them the additional comfort of knowing their estate will be used for worthy purposes when they no longer need it. Setting up a scholarship plan for needy students, nursing scholarships, mental health funds, or church memorials are common.

One warning. Wills need to be kept up to date. I have seen far too many elderly patients die, and their wills are out of date. The people named in their wills may no longer be alive, or circumstances may have changed greatly. I took care of one lady whose will gave all her possessions to a granddaughter who had been close to her when the granddaughter was young. However, when my patient became older, the granddaughter had abandoned her, had gotten mixed up with drugs, and was living with a boyfriend in parts unknown. For several years, all of the care my patient required was done by friends and neighbors who were very generous and comforting to her. She expressed a desire to reward these wonderful people for their care, but forgot to change the will. At her death, the verbal plans meant nothing. The granddaughter did not even attend the funeral, but did swing into town long enough to pick up the inheritance check, before disappearing again. There was not even a "thank you" to those who had labored so long caring for my patient.

One Vintage Lady I know tells me she updates her will every year at Christmas time. "Earlier," she says, "I planned to leave everything to my husband. I outlived him, so I changed it to my children. They are all doing well now on their own, so I've decided to leave them enough to remember me by, but I have decided to set up a fund through my church to help any student that decides to study for the ministry. My minister has helped me so much, and it gives me a warm feeling to think that I can be helping other people like myself, perhaps generations from now, because I helped educate a young minister."

Writing a will should be a positive experience. Vintage People have learned to use the reality of death to enhance their lives in the moment, as well as helping in the future. Bequests are not whimsical, but reflect the reality of life that Vintage People deal with in a positive and creative way.

Dying itself is not only accepted, but often looked at in a positive vein as well. In a letter, dated February 12, 1756, Benjamin Franklin attempted to console a friend who had lost a loved one. It expresses a great truth about death that I have found to be the philosophy of many Vintage People. He wrote: "That bodies should be lent us is a kind and benevolent act of God. When they become unfit for these purposes and afford us pain instead of pleasure—instead of an aid, become an encumbrance and answer none of the intentions for which they were given—it is equally kind and benevolent that a way is provided by which we may get rid of them. Death is that way."

Vintage People recognize death as an intimate milestone that is a natural progression of life. They plan for it and recognize their own mortality, accepting facts they cannot change. Most Vintage People even look forward to a transformation and continued eternal life. Winston Churchill once said, "I am ready to meet my Maker. Whether my Maker is prepared for the ordeal of meeting me is another matter."

I love the comment by the evangelist Dwight L. Moody when asked about dying. His reply was, "Some day you will read in the papers that D. L. Moody of East Northfield is dead. Don't you believe a word of it! At that moment I shall be more alive than I am now. I shall have gone up higher, that is all—out of this old clay tenement into a house that is immortal; a body that death cannot touch, that sin cannot taint, a body fashioned like unto His glorious body."

What a glorious future we have when it is viewed in this manner. Vintage People view death as an important part of living. How would our lives be upon this planet if we knew we would never die? We would definitely not be human. Billy Graham says, "The fact is, we cannot truly face life until we have learned to face the fact that it will be taken away from us." There is power in accepting our mortality.

James Weldon Johnson, author of *God's Trombones— Seven Negro Sermons in Verse,* beautifully summarizes death in this excerpt of a funeral sermon:

> "While we were watching round her bed,
> She turned her eyes and looked away,
> She saw what we couldn't see;
> She saw Old Death. She saw Old Death
> Coming like a falling star.
> But Death didn't frighten Sister Caroline;
> He looked to her a welcome friend.
> And she whispered to us: 'I'm going home',
> And she smiled and closed her eyes."

SIXTEEN

PEARLS

"For wisdom is better than jewels, and all that you
may desire cannot compare with her."
—Proverbs 8:11

In medical school we treasured "pearls," the small, rich, practical bits of wisdom and information that the most respected attending physicians cast before us lowly students. Pearls were facts and pieces of advice learned by experience and not written anywhere in the standard medical textbooks. They were valuable and unique.

Likewise, I have gathered many "pearls" from the interviews and many years of medical practice in dealing with Vintage People. Some have already been suggested earlier in this book; some have not. I want to list many of these "pearls" so that we can all use them to our advantage as we live life and work toward becoming Vintage People.

"Don't ever dress old. If you dress old, you feel old. But don't dress too young either. Then people will just laugh at you for trying to be what you are not, and you will feel old again."

"Sing often!"

"Keep up on current events. It helps to know what is going on around you, and it keeps you from living in the past."

"Get a pet!"

"Read! Reading keeps the mind young."

"Don't ever give in to aches and pains. I figure I'm going to hurt about as much while I'm out and going as if I'm sitting at home thinking about how much I hurt."

"Trust God."

"Don't ever use segregation, racism or color as an excuse."

"Find a doctor you trust, and follow his advice. There are a lot of miracles of modern medicine that can help. For example, I finally gave in and got a hearing aid—it changed my life around."

"Always be courteous. Some older people tend to lose their inhibitions and become rude. That never helps, and just makes you feel worse too."

"Work hard—it's good for you!"

"Don't always talk about the past. Don't start every sentence with, 'When I was your age,' or 'I can remember when....' That dates you, and most younger people don't want to hear it anyway."

"Appreciate your spouse and your friends."

"Be flexible. Don't lecture young people about their life-styles. If you always criticize, they will just stay away from you and not want to share with you."

"Spend time with children. I always feel energized when I have spent time with children."

"Keep a lot of love in your life."

"Being successful and living long is 199 percent attitude. I have discovered that most all of my success has come from how I felt from the neck up."

"Serve others."

"Don't ever retire—just change careers. Having something to do adds worth to our lives. We need to feel like we are accomplishing something every day."

"Don't feel sorry for yourself. When bad things happen, refuse to join the 'pity me club.'"

"Travel as much as possible."

"Don't worry about money—things usually take care of themselves if you just do what you really like doing; and do it well."

"Accept the fact that you are aging and use it to your advantage."

"Be independent when you can—but don't be too stubborn to accept help when you need it."

"Be silly."

"Start each day well. Get up and get dressed for the day—you will feel better."

"Practice what you preach."

"Go to clown school."

"Spend time with family; children, grandchildren, extended family, and with friends."

"Have faith in God, compassion for all people, and spend time with church work and volunteer service."

"Have an optimistic, hopeful attitude and a sense of humor."

"Know what you stand for, and why."

"Learn as much as you can about yourself—it is easier to develop compassion for others if we trust ourselves."

"Establish daily routines."

"Smile a lot—even when you don't feel like it."

"Do things that make you feel good."

"Write letters to people and to companies. It is amazing what you can do by writing letters."

"Listen to yourself. Don't rely upon others—you are usually right."

"When bad things happen, just say to yourself: 'Life is teaching me!' Use this and you will see things much differently."

"Be honest with yourself. If you don't want to do something, like exercise, don't make up excuses. Just say you don't like to do it!"

"Work hard. People who work hard are less tired than those that sit around all day."

"Look a situation over. Then make a decision and stick to it."

"Be sure to enjoy what you have."

"Don't be afraid of mistakes."

"Always exceed the expectations of your job—even if you are doing volunteer work, and even if no one will notice."

"Always have goals to pursue."

"Remember in life that you always have a choice in your attitude. Events, governments, and other people can control external circumstances, but you can always control your attitude."

APPENDIX

Florence's story

An eighty-one-year-old Vintage Lady named Florence sent me such a beautiful description of all the characteristics we have talked about in this book that I have included it here in its entirety as an example of where we can all end up in life if we follow the characteristics and power of Vintage People. I look forward to being like Florence when I am her age.

Dear Jerry,

I have been invited to make a professional video tape about "Attitude for Seniors." This will be made in Florida. I want to thank you for your challenging letter. It made me pull out the notes I had made.

I know I'm sending way too much, but I hope you can glean from them my feelings about aging. If I had to sum it up I would say: attitude is developmental, faith in God, yourself, and your world is number one, and you must have three philosophies —life, health, and relationships. I have made comments on each. I apologize for sending so much, but at this point, I can't dilute it.

One of the best examples of living life to its fullest came from you at Toastmasters club. It was the time you showed "slides" of your visit to the zoo—only the slides were pretend. You put it on a blank wall, and it was a blank picture! You and I were the only ones to see the monkeys, the giraffes, and the excitement. The rest of the people saw only a blank wall. I saw my philosophy of life come alive—going beyond the edge of the familiar, my belief in expectations, the need to focus, and the joy in humor. Believe me, any attitude on aging is developmental. Thanks for giving me that little demonstration.

Long before retirement you must decide on these two things: What you want to *do*, and what you want to *be*. Adolescence has no corner on these two questions. It has nothing to do with a career or lifestyle—it's *you* at the center.

As aging becomes a reality, I believe each person must have three philosophies of life. They must be your own—not the ones your mother taught you, or from church, or the Boy Scouts. A philosophy you can speak right up and claim. You must have one about life, one about health, and one about relationships.

Life: Each day go beyond the edge of the familiar. You can do this in a wheelchair, a hands on situation, or in a research lab. Do it!

Health: Discipline is the key word. It has to be both inside and outside of your body. If you walk, drink water, do deep breathing, take pills—do it regularly. Discipline!

Relationships: Don't try to change anyone. Learn the power of motivation and how it works.

After you have your philosophies, get them so ingrained in your body, mind and soul that you can have some fun. Study expectations, yours as well as others. When you are waiting for the elevator—what do you expect? Do you expect to wait ten minutes, that there will be people on the elevator that you don't like, or the thing will stop in mid air? Your attitude about life develops from your expectations.

I have a friend who says, "I'm going to make the most out of what I have left." Wrong! I beg her to leave off the word "left!" Tacking that word on to her philosophy sends a message to me. She has lost something, or she isn't as good as she should be. Let her say, "I'm going to make the most of what I have!"

Start your day—YOU start it! Get up and be dressed by eight a.m. Have makeup and shoes on. Make your bed so you can't crawl back into it. You can rest later if you must. Be ready to meet a friend for coffee. Be ready for the day!

Eat correctly. Don't stand at the refrigerator and have your lunch. Don't eat in segments. Plan, prepare, and eat in a complete dining atmosphere. Put a little fun thing in front of your plate. Put a smile thing on your table.

Follow through on your ideas. Don't let the idea of exercise die at the coffee table. I have a small trampoline. I checked it out with my doctor. It is wonderful, with no hard impact on the body. Let an idea become a reality.

Have faith in God. This is rule number one. I firmly believe that God is in the midst of me. I listen, I meditate, I am lead.

Focus on your strengths. It may be your smile, your ability to sing, or to encourage others. I belong to the Chamber of Commerce; I read the daily papers and do not dwell on the obituaries or the hospital notes.

Be careful of your appearance. Get a younger person to check you out. Enhance yourself. If you have to wear old lady shoes, wear them with the assurance that they are right for balance and safety. Don't let them determine your mood. If you have to carry a cane, do it as though it is an accessory like glasses or a hearing aid. Simply know that it makes you more effective.

Experience life! Experience life as it is *today*. I entered a three-mile marathon. I was the last one in by the time limit. It was not competition or being a show off. It was feeling wonderful within my limits. People clapped for the last one in as well as the first. Not for being old or young, but because of being a part of the total experience.

Plan ahead! Seven years before I retired I made this list of what I wanted to *be,* and what I wanted to *do:*

What I want to do:
  I want to bring happiness to others.
  I want to motivate others.
  I want to have a business of my own.
  I want everything that a happy couple would have
      after retirement—home, travel, financial security,
      ability to cope.
  I want to maintain my sense of humor.
  I want to maintain my good health.
  I want to believe in Divine Guidance.
What I want to be:
  Flexible in mind and body.
  Happy from the inside.
  To be recognized as a radiant Christian.
  I want to understand myself and others.

I want to be loving with all of its meanings—generous, kind, etc.

At eighty-one years old, I have accomplished most of these:

> I am a professional Christian Clown.
> I am a certified Reflexologist and have a good business.
> I have excellent health.
> I winter in Florida each year.
> God is my source.
> I am up and dressed every morning.

I must have a sense of humor or I would never attempted this reflection on aging—I would have been playing bridge or doing my woodcarving.

Accomplishment did not develop during a specific age span—attitude, curiosity, humor, and self-confidence has not only been my life-style—it was my inheritance.

—Submitted by
Florence Goforth Stephens